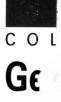

C O L

Ge

Ian A. R. More BSc PhD MD FRCPath

Senior Lecturer in Pathology, University of Glasgow
Honorary Consultant Pathologist,
Western Infirmary, Glasgow

Ian L. Brown BSc MB ChB MRCPath

Lecturer in Pathology, University of Glasgow
Honorary Consultant Pathologist,
Western Infirmary, Glasgow

D0309710

Churchill Livingstone

EDINBURGH LONDON MADRID MELBOURNE NEW YORK AND TOKYO 1994

2 8 MAR 2004

CHURCHILL LIVINGSTONE
Medical Division of Longman Group UK Limited

Distributed in the United States of America by
Churchill Livingstone Inc., 650 Avenue of the Americas,
New York, N.Y. 10011, and by associated companies,
branches and representatives throughout the world.

© Longman Group UK Limited 1994

First published as Colour Aids—General Pathology 1991
    Reprinted 1994

ISBN 0-443-04949-1

British Library Cataloguing in Publication Data
A catalogue record for this book is available from the
British Library.

Library of Congress Cataloging in Publication Data
A catalogue record for this book is available from the
Library of Congress.

25/7/97

M

Publisher
Timothy Horne

Project Editor
Jim Killgore

Production
Nancy Arnott

Designer
Design Resources Unit

Sales Promotion Executive
Marion Pollock

The
publisher's
policy is to use
**paper manufactured
from sustainable forests**

Printed in Hong Kong
GC/02

Preface

This short volume in the Colour Guides series provides short notes and colour illustrations on general pathological processes. As such it will be of value to medical students in their undergraduate courses in pathology and also to medical practitioners preparing for post graduate examinations in surgery, medicine, obstetrics and gynaecology. It will also prove useful to students in related fields such as nursing, speech therapy, medical laboratory scientific officers and medical physics who are expected to have a basic understanding of the processes of disease.

Glasgow   I.L.B.
1994   I.A.R.M.

Contents

1 / Necrosis

Definition Necrosis is the death of cells or groups of cells which are still part of the living body.

Aetiology Necrosis may be caused by a variety of insults:
- The decrease in the blood supply to an area of tissue may cause its death. For example, myocardial infarction occurs when an atheromatous-based thrombotic occlusion of a branch of the coronary artery leads to the death of that portion of cardiac muscle supplied by the vessel (Fig. 1).
- Toxins (organic compounds derived from a variety of animal, plant, insect and bacterial sources) can cause cell death. For example lecithinase produced by *Cl. welchi* degrades cell membranes which then rupture.
- Immunological injury in the form of hypersensitivity reactions (Fig. 2) gives rise to injury by the reaction of complement activation products or T-lymphocytes with specific sites on the cell surface.
- Cellular disruption due to the intracellular growth of an organism is a cause of cell death, e.g. the typical cold sore due to herpes simplex virus.
- Physical damage can be incurred in a number of ways:
  —mechanical trauma disrupts cell membranes and organelles
  —heat increases the rate at which proteins and enzymes are denatured
  —freezing of tissues gives rise to the formation of ice crystals within the cellular compartments with resultant mechanical disruption.

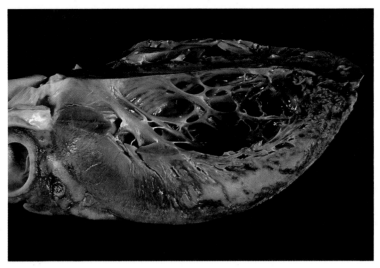

Fig. 1 Coronary artery thrombosis with associated myocardial infarction.

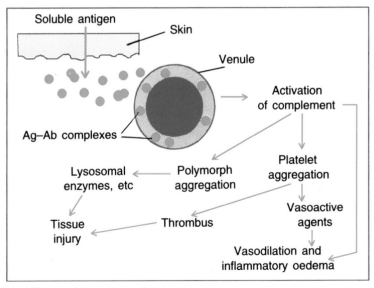

Fig. 2 Diagram of the Arthus reaction.

General appearance The appearance of dead tissue varies according to the type of tissue involved and the nature of the aetiological agent. There are four main appearances.

Coagulative necrosis
This is seen best in solid tissues, e.g. in the kidney (Fig. 3). After 12 to 24 hours the dead tissue has a yellowish/white colour, is swollen and has a firm texture. It rapidly develops a red rim, indicating an inflammatory reaction. The dead tissue is removed and scarring takes place (p. 47).

Microscopic appearance. The nuclei of the dead cells become shrunken and dense (*pyknosis*), break up into discrete clumps of chromatin (*karyorrhexis*) or dissolve (*karyolysis*). In haematoxylin and eosin stained sections the ghost outlines of the dead cells remain but the cytoplasm becomes swollen and granular. It takes up more of the eosin and is often strikingly pink. Enzyme activity is lost in the dead tissue— succinic dehydrogenase is particularly rapidly affected and is used as a test of viability.

Colliquative necrosis
Colliquative necrosis occurs in tissues with a high water content. In cerebral infarction (Fig. 4) the necrotic brain tissue becomes soft and eventually breaks down completely to form a cyst filled with turbid fluid. The dead cells absorb water and finally disintegrate with complete loss of architecture.

Caseation
This is a form of necrosis in which there is total loss of architecture (Fig. 5). The tissue becomes soft and crumbly and has the texture of cottage cheese.

Microscopic appearance. This shows loss of cellular outline; the caseous material has an amorphous, eosinophilic appearance.

Gangrene
This occurs in necrotic skin (Fig. 6) or mucosa invaded by microorganisms. The tissues are discoloured due to deposition of sulphides derived from haemoglobin, and foul smelling (*putrefaction*) due to the production of hydrogen sulphide gas.

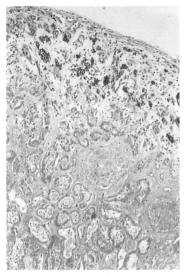

Fig. 3 Infarct of kidney.

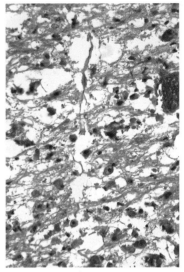

Fig. 4 Cerebral infarct.

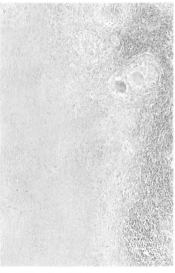

Fig. 5 Caseation in tuberculous lymph node.

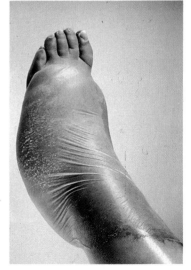

Fig. 6 Venous gangrene.

Autolysis

Mechanism   The changes of necrosis occur largely as a result of liberation of lytic enzymes by cells. These enzymes are normally kept in an inactive form in lysosomes. In necrotic cells anaerobic glycolysis lowers the pH, activating acid hydrolases. The release of phosphatases and proteolytic enzymes also degrades membranes and causes lysosomal breakdown. A large number of small molecules are produced raising cellular osmotic pressure and drawing water into the dying cell, which swells. Heat or chemical damage may cause protein denaturation but autolysis will not develop as enzymes are inactivated. Some of the changes in necrotic tissue are due to enzymes from neutrophils and macrophages attracted into the dead tissue. It takes time for these changes to develop and this explains the delay before necrosis becomes evident.

Sequelae   The effects of necrosis vary according to the size and type of tissue involved:
- loss of the spleen is consistent with long life
- loss of a small portion of the conducting system of the heart may be fatal
- a kidney may be donated indicating a redundancy of at least 50% in renal tissue
- the loss of brain tissue is irreversible (Fig. 7)
- the liver is rapidly reconstituted after a partial hepatectomy.

Tissue death leads to the liberation of a variety of salts and macromolecules into the circulation producing nonspecific effects (e.g. fever). Other effects may be relatively specific for the type of tissue damaged. Aminotransferases are released from an area of myocardial infarction—these enzymes may be utilized in diagnosis and assessment (Fig. 8).

Loss of function of necrotic tissue may have important consequences for tissues remote from the site of injury. Loss of hormones after injury to an endocrine gland will lead to atrophy of the target tissue.

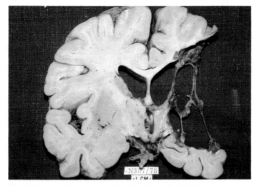

Fig. 7 Apoplectic cyst at site of old cerebral infarct.

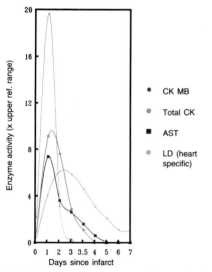

- ● CK MB
- ● Total CK
- ■ AST
- ● LD (heart specific)

Fig. 8 Release of cardiac enzymes after an episode of infarction.

Apoptosis

Definition This is the programmed (active) self-destruction of cells. The death of cells may be physiological and is an essential component of cell turnover, where cell death is matched with regeneration. RNA and protein synthesis and a supply of ATP are necessary for apoptosis.

The cell programmed for destruction shrinks and condenses, fragments and is ingested by neighbouring cells. The ingested fragments appear as lysosomal vacuoles and are referred to as apoptotic vesicles or bodies (Figs 9 & 10).

Occurrence Active cell destruction is found in the gastrointestinal tract, the skin, the haemopoietic system and in endocrine-dependent involution. It is also responsible for programmed destruction of cells (e.g. in the interdigital clefts) during embryonic development. The process does not invoke an inflammatory reaction.

Apoptosis may also occur pathologically. Councilman bodies in the liver are the result of cell-mediated immune responses to altered hepatocytes infected by hepatitis B virus. It is also prominent in damage following radiation exposure, and accounts for the loss of cell numbers which occurs in pathological atrophy.

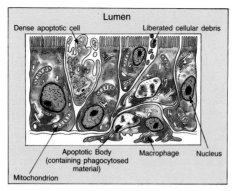

Fig. 9 Diagram of apoptosis.

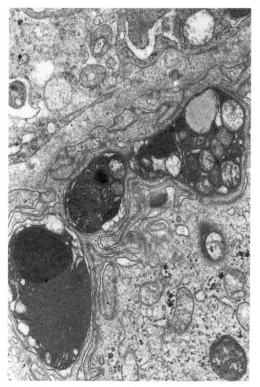

Fig. 10 Electron micrograph of apoptotic bodies in human endometrium.

2 / Non-lethal cell damage

Cells possess very efficient repair mechanisms. In many cells damage does not lead to necrosis, but to deficiencies within the cell and in interactions with other cells. Mild defects will only be demonstrated by electron microscopy.

Ultrastructure Membranes delimit the various intracellular compartments and aid in enzyme reactions by bringing reactants into close spatial relation. The following illustrate clinical conditions in which ultrastructural changes have been identified:

- In hereditary spherocytosis, a disorder of red cell membranes, there is increased membrane permeability to salts, an increased activity of the Na^+ pump and accelerated phospholipid metabolism. Because of the loss of lipid there is diminished surface area and cell volume approaches that of a sphere (Fig. 11).
- Anoxia and some poisons result in disaggregation of ribosomes, loss of parallel arrays and vacuolation of the endoplasmic reticulum.
- Mitochondria are the site of oxidative phosphorylation. With decreased concentration of O_2 there is decreased ATP and the Na^+ pump becomes less efficient. Mitochondria swell and the result is called 'cloudy swelling' (Fig. 12).
- Lytic enzymes are packaged in lysosomes, which can be damaged by some bacteria and hypervitaminosis A. In silicosis, macrophages ingest silica and convert it to silicic acid which causes rupture by binding to lysosomal phospholipid. Some photosensitivity reactions, e.g. in porphyria, involve destabilization of the lysosome. In diseases characterized by lack of specific lysosomal enzymes, macromolecules accumulate and cannot be degraded further within the lysosomes. In Fabry's disease, an X-linked disorder, glycosphingolipids accumulate within endothelial and smooth muscle cells due to a deficiency of an alphagalactosidase. Death usually results between 35 and 45 years from cardiac or renal failure (Figs 13 & 14).

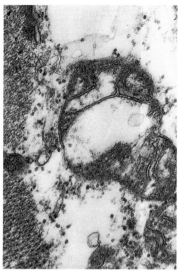

Fig. 11 Blood film showing scattered spherocytes.

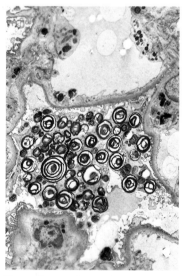

Fig. 12 Electron micrograph of vacuolated mitochondria.

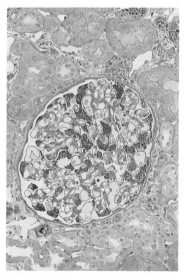

Fig. 13 Glomerulus in Fabry's disease (PAS stain).

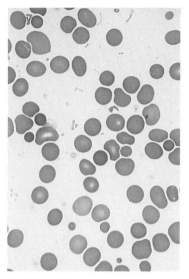

Fig. 14 Electron micrograph of inclusions in Fabry's disease.

Fatty change

Definition The result of an imbalance between the amount of fat and fatty acids entering a cell and their rate of utilization.

Cells accumulating lipid are injured. The liver has a central role in fat metabolism and is most commonly affected (Fig. 15). Small droplets of triglyceride accumulate in the cell cytoplasm. These usually remain small and discrete although they may fuse to form globules filling the cell (Fig. 16). Perivenular hepatocytes are usually affected first.

Aetiology Fatty change may be caused by hypoxia (e.g. chronic anaemia, congestive heart failure), starvation or wasting diseases.

Pathological obesity

In a small proportion of individuals obesity is related to abnormalities of the hypothalamus, giving rise to deficient pituitary secretion and to adiposity associated with failure of sexual development. Deficiencies of thyroid secretion may play a part.

Metabolic disorders

• Storage of complex lipids may occur secondary to lysosomal enzyme deficiency, e.g. Gaucher's disease.
• In familial hyperbeta-lipoproteinaemia there is a huge increase in the plasma lipoprotein due to a lack of the appropriate low density lipoprotein (LDL) receptor (Fig. 17). Cholesterol is also raised. Such patients suffer from atheroma at an early age and may develop xanthomas in skin, tendons, etc.
• Deficiency of the enzymes responsible for depolymerizing glycogen gives rise to excess glycogen storage, e.g. Von Gierke's disease.
• In Pompe's disease the glycogen accumulates secondary to a deficiency of lysosomal glucosidase.

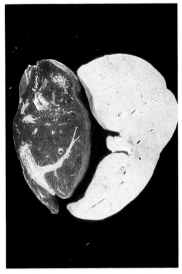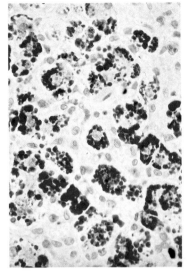

Fig. 15 Fatty liver with normal liver for comparison.

Fig. 16 Fatty liver (Oil red O stain).

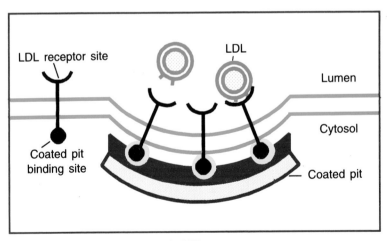

Fig. 17 Diagram of low density lipoprotein (LDL) receptor.

3 / Cell damage by ionizing radiation

Aetiology Cell damage can be caused by:
- X-rays and gamma-rays
- electrons, protons and neutrons.

Damage depends on other conditions during irradiation, e.g. oxygen potentiates the effects.

Figure 18 shows the relative annual dose of radiation (in grays) to the UK population. It is interesting to note that preventable radiation is responsible for only 1.5% of exposure. In some geographical areas radon presents a significant risk.

Tissues vary in their sensitivity to radiation. Tissues with a high cell turnover are most susceptible to radiation damage, e.g. skin, gastrointestinal tract, bone marrow, malignant tumours. The ability of cells to multiply is decreased and there is a drop in cell numbers; the surviving cells divide and the deficit is eventually made good. The rate at which this happens depends on the percentage of surviving cells and the rate of division. If the cell population falls below a critical level the tissue may lose its functional effectiveness.

Damaged cells may make abortive attempts to divide giving rise to bizarre cytological appearances. Some cells may show little effect; however, damage will have been sustained and may become apparent when the cells divide. There is therefore no safe lower limit for radiation damage.

Microscopic appearance The appearance depends on the type, total dose and rate of irradiation. In the skin the following changes occur:
- blood vessels dilate and there is acute inflammation
- mitotic activity is arrested in the basal layer
- blood vessel walls are infiltrated by fibrin (Fig. 19)
- the intima proliferates giving an 'onion skin' appearance
- bizarre fibroblast nuclei appear in the dermis (Fig. 20).

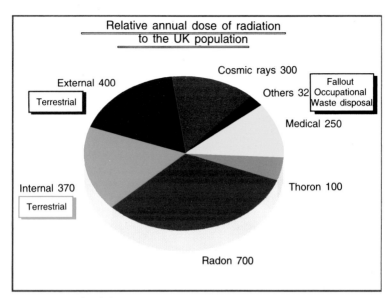

Fig. 18 Sources of radiation.

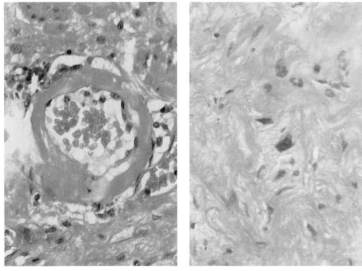

Fig. 19 Radiation changes in blood vessels.

Fig. 20 Radiation changes in fibroblasts.

4 / Atrophy

Definition   Atrophy is diminution in size of a cell or reduction in the essential tissue of an organ due to decrease in the size or number of its specialized cells.

Physiological atrophy occurs with age, affecting all cells. Atrophic cells lose their specialized functions and may accumulate a yellow/brown pigment (*lipofuscin*—see p. 87) (Fig. 21).

Aetiology   Atrophy may be caused by defective nutrition. In starvation there is a loss of fat and cells. There may also be a toxic element as in the cachexia of malignant disease.

Localized nutritional deficiency results from poor blood supply, e.g. secondary to arterial disease. Disuse atrophy occurs when there is diminished functional activity; e.g. muscle around a joint which has been immobilized loses bulk, and there may be loss of calcium from bones in prolonged bed rest. Such changes are usually reversible.

Interference with the nerve supply causes degeneration in the muscle supplied, e.g. after destruction of the spinal cord anterior horn cells in polio. These changes are irreversible (Fig. 22).

Some tissues require hormone stimulation for their continued function; in its absence the tissue atrophies, e.g. damage to the pituitary may cause atrophy of the thyroid which in turn may cause atrophy of the skin.

Toxic atrophy, such as muscle wasting in fevers, is secondary to increased catabolism of protein.

When a tumour or cyst presses on an organ, interference with the blood supply results in pressure atrophy.

In Alzheimer's disease cerebral tissue atrophies as a result of loss of neurones (Fig. 23).

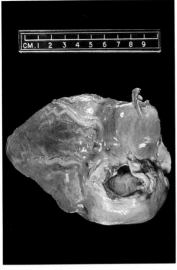

Fig. 21 Atrophic heart showing loss of fat (brown atrophy).

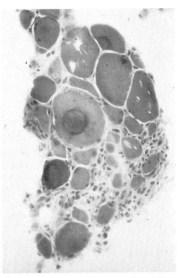

Fig. 22 Patchy atrophy of skeletal muscle fibres.

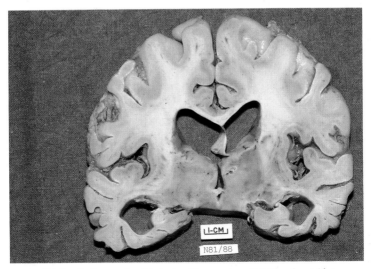

Fig. 23 Alzheimer's disease. Atrophic brain with secondary dilatation of ventricles.

5 / Metaplasia

Definition Metaplasia is a cellular response to injury in which one type of differentiated epithelium is transformed into another.

Aetiology Cigarette smoking causes the pseudostratified columnar, ciliated epithelium of the bronchus to change to stratified squamous epithelium. In the salivary ducts, gall bladder, renal pelvis and urinary bladder the presence of stones (Fig. 24) also causes the mucosa to change to stratified squamous epithelium which is more able to withstand the insult. In the prostate following treatment with oestrogens for prostatic carcinoma there may be squamous metaplasia of the ductal epithelium (Fig. 25).

Many stimuli which give rise to metaplasia may also result in neoplasia. In the example above cigarette smoking gives rise to metaplasia which may progressively evolve through dysplasia (p. 97) into neoplasia—resulting in squamous carcinoma of the bronchus.

Metaplasia may be found in or close to neoplastic tissue. For example in autoimmune chronic gastritis the gastric mucosa loses its specialized chief and parietal cells which are replaced by Paneth cells, tall columnar cells and goblet cells—intestinal metaplasia (Fig. 26). This metaplastic change has been proposed as a premalignant phase in some types of gastric carcinoma. However, it may merely represent an epiphenomenon in mucosa adjacent to the tumour.

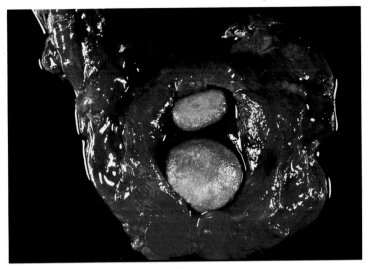

Fig. 24 Bladder stones in an inflamed bladder.

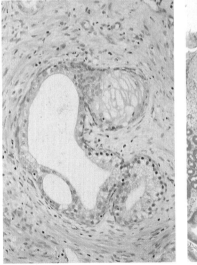

Fig. 25 Squamous metaplasia in the prostate.

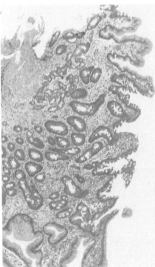

Fig. 26 Intestinal metaplasia in the stomach.

6 / Inflammation

Inflammation is the response of living tissue to injury, which may be due to microorganisms, immunological mechanisms, release of substances from necrotic tissue, radiation, extremes of temperature, trauma, chemicals and toxins.

Pus is a creamy yellow fluid consisting of living, dying and dead neutrophil polymorphs, organisms, and dead and damaged cells suspended in inflammatory exudate (Fig. 27).

Inflammatory cells

Neutrophil polymorphs (Fig. 27)
• Characteristic cells of acute inflammation.
• First to arrive at the site of injury.
• Enzymatically and phagocytically active.
• Active in hypoxic conditions.
• Respond to chemotaxis.

Macrophages
• Derived from blood monocytes.
• Migrate through venules to inflamed tissue.
• Become activated macrophages in tissues.
• Actively phagocytic.

Eosinophil polymorphs (Fig. 28)
• Involved in hypersensitivity reactions.
• Release aryl sulphatase, histaminase.
• Associated with parasitic infections.

Plasma cells (Fig. 29)
• Stimulated B-lymphocytes, produce antibody.
• Chronic inflammatory cells.
• Appear after 1 week.

Lymphocytes (Fig. 30)
• Non-suppurative chronic inflammation.
• T-lymphocytes responsible for release of lymphokines which attract other cells; also involved in control of B-lymphocytes.

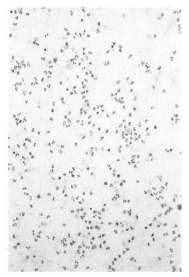

Fig. 27 Neutrophil polymorphonuclear leucocytes from pus.

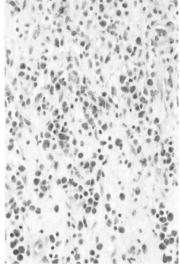

Fig. 28 Eosinophil polymorphonuclear leucocytes from a nasal polyp.

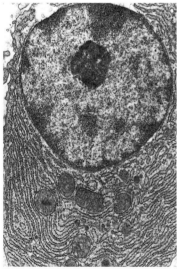

Fig. 29 Electron micrograph of plasma cell.

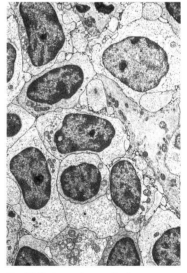

Fig. 30 Electron micrograph of lymphocytes.

7 / Acute inflammatory reaction

Definition The acute inflammatory reaction occurs in the first few hours after injury. It is characterized by changes in the microcirculation and by emigration and accumulation of polymorphs.

Clinical features The cardinal signs of inflammation are:
- *rubor* (redness): due to dilatation of small blood vessels (Fig. 31)
- *calor* (heat): felt in superficial tissues due to increased blood flow
- *dolor* (pain): due to the release of chemical mediators and to local pressure effects
- *tumor* (swelling): due to local oedema (Figs 32 & 33)
- *loss of function*: a complex response to the other features.

The vascular response The inflammatory exudate responsible for local swelling is the result of increased vascular permeability. There are two major causes:
- Chemical mediators such as histamine and bradykinin cause an immediate increase in permeability lasting up to 15 minutes, due to the formation of gaps between endothelial cells of small veins and venules.
- Longer periods of leakiness are usually the result of tissue damage, and if sustained may indicate endothelial disruption. Minor damage may give short-lived changes.

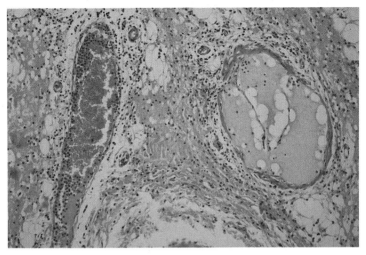

Fig. 31 Dilated vascular channels in acute inflammation.

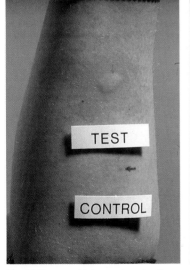

Fig. 32 Hypersensitivity reaction showing local oedema.

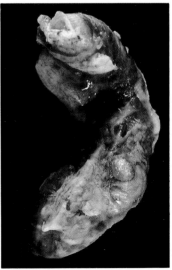

Fig. 33 Perforated acute appendicitis with vascular congestion and a fibrinous exudate.

The
inflammatory
exudate

The inflammatory exudate formed as a consequence of the increased vascular permeability (Fig. 34) consists of a high turnover pool of protein-rich (35–50 g/l) fluid, containing plasma proteins, particularly fibrinogen. Small blood vessel walls act as filters and molecules move by passive diffusion or bulk transfer. Some endothelia are fenestrated and allow free movement; others are continuous and less permeable.

Emigration of
polymorphs

The emigration of leucocytes is complex, involving vascular changes and chemotaxis.

- 'Pavementing' of leucocytes occurs in venules and is the first step in emigration. Damaged endothelium becomes sticky and leucocytes adhere to its surface giving the appearance of pavementing or margination (Fig. 35).
- Leucocyte emigration follows by active amoeboid movement of the pavemented leucocytes through the vessel wall. They infiltrate between cell junctions, which then reform behind the emigrated cell. The basement membrane is penetrated by the cell, and then reseals (Fig. 36).
- Chemotaxis is the process by which the leucocyte is attracted along a concentration gradient of a chemotactic agent such as complement factors (C5a, or C567), lymphokines, eosinophil chemotactic factor of anaphylaxis (ECFA), and leukotriene (LTB4).
- Chemical mediators released from damaged tissue are responsible for many of the features of the acute inflammatory reaction. The chemicals involved include kinins, complement factors, plasmin, histamine, serotonin, prostaglandins and leukotrienes.

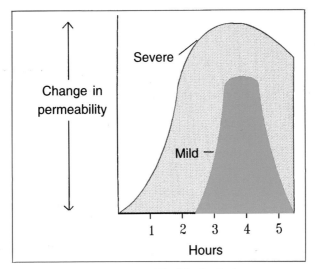

Fig. 34 Diagram of vascular permeability following insult.

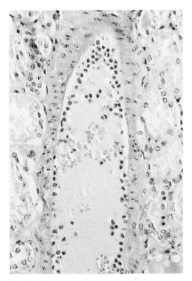

Fig. 35 Margination of neutrophil polymorphs.

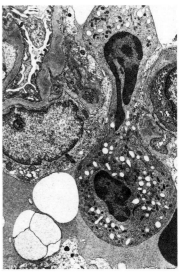

Fig. 36 Emigration of neutrophil polymorph between the endothelial cells in a glomerular capillary.

Advantageous effects The removal of dead tissue and foreign material and the inactivation and dilution of toxins are the main effects of inflammation.

Phagocytosis. Leucocytes are responsible for phagocytosis.

- Plasma protein coats the target particle (opsonization) enhancing adhesion of the particle to the phagocytic cell (Fig. 37A). Specific lgG class antibodies, activated third component of complement (C3b) and its inactivated form (C3bi), and plasma fibronectin are the major opsonins. There are specific receptors for each of these three groups.
- The opsonized particle is then enveloped by cytoplasm and included in a phagocytic vacuole (Fig. 37B) which fuses with a lysosome.
- The ingested material undergoes digestion (Fig. 38) as a result of the action of numerous lysosomal hydrolases which are optimally active at a low pH.

Microbial killing by this means is relatively inefficient, and the disposal of microorganisms is due to the production of H_2O_2 and free radicals. These moieties are produced during the respiratory burst which follows activation of cell membrane NADPH oxidase by phagocytosis.

Inflammatory exudate. The inflammatory exudate is high in fibrinogen which is converted to a fibrin meshwork under the action of thromboplastin (Fig. 39). This meshwork inhibits the movement of organisms and gives phagocytes a supporting structure.

The fluid also acts as a diluent for toxins, delivers antibodies and nutrients to the damaged tissue, and carries antigenic material to the draining lymph nodes.

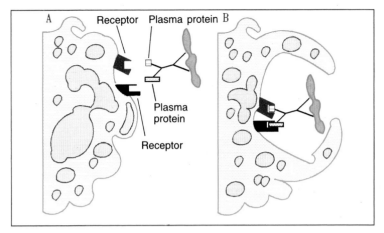

Fig. 37 Diagram of opsonization.

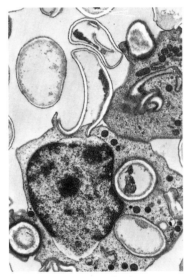

Fig. 38 Electron micrograph of macrophages ingesting zymosan granules.

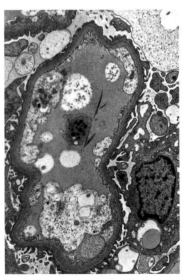

Fig. 39 Electron micrograph of fibrin and platelets in glomerular capillary.

Harmful effects   Acutely inflamed tissues swell with resultant disruption of their physiological function. For example:
- laryngeal oedema may give rise to stridor due to obstruction of the airways
- in the cranial cavity swelling will result in raised intracranial pressure which may cause pressure necrosis of brain tissue or nerves, coma and eventually death
- in osteomyelitis the increased pressure in the medullary cavity may cause secondary bone necrosis
- in severe cystitis there is pain and frequency of micturition (Fig. 40)
- gastric ulcers give dyspepsia, and bleed resulting in iron deficiency anaemia and/or haematemesis (Fig. 41).

In some cases the inflammatory reaction may be inappropriate, e.g. in hay fever, conjunctivitis and rhinitis following exposure to grass pollens.

Sequelae   The process of acute inflammation may follow a number of paths.

Resolution. This means restoration of the tissue to normality. It is the usual result of mild inflammation due to physical or chemical agents, or to infections which do not result in necrosis. Necrotic tissue is replaced by fibrosis which results in scar formation rendering resolution impossible.

Suppuration. This is usually caused by infection with pyogenic organisms (Fig. 42) such as *Staphylococcus aureus*, *Streptococcus pyogenes*, the gonococcus and the meningococcus.

Pus may form diffusely in tissue planes or may collect in discrete foci—abscesses, which may rupture releasing the pus. Once empty the abscess walls adhere to one another, firstly by fibrin then by granulation tissue. Fibrinous exudates on free surfaces result in fibrous adhesions, e.g. between loops of bowel (Fig. 43).

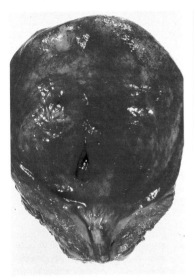

Fig. 40 Severe acute cystitis.

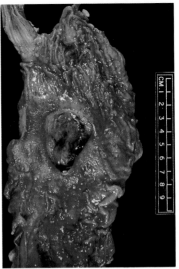

Fig. 41 Large benign gastric ulcer.

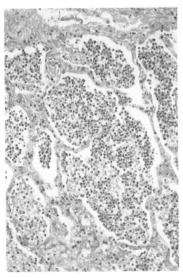

Fig. 42 Pneumonia.

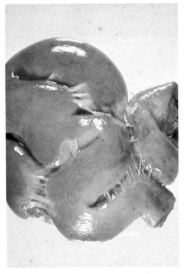

Fig. 43 Fibrous adhesions between loops of small bowel following peritonitis.

8 / Chronic inflammatory reaction

Definition   Any prolonged inflammatory reaction is termed chronic.

Types   There are two main types:
- following on from an acute inflammatory reaction
- showing chronic inflammatory changes from the beginning.

Aetiology   Suppurative acute inflammation may progress to chronic inflammation usually due to a failure to drain the pus or because of the presence of foreign material or necrotic tissue.

Chronic inflammatory disease from the outset is usually attributable to:

- The nature of the insult, e.g. asbestos, talc.
- Inadequate tissue response, e.g. due to poor blood supply.
- Disturbed immune response, e.g. rheumatoid arthritis (Fig. 44).
- Certain microorganisms, e.g. *Mycobacterium tuberculosis*, produce a chronic inflammatory response from the outset. The disease is characterized by the production of multiple granulomas in various organs, e.g. in lung (Fig. 45). Where the granulomas become confluent there is formation of central 'cheese-like' necrosis—caseation (Fig. 46). The mycobacteria are identified in tissue sections by the Ziehl–Neelsen stain which exploits the chemical characteristics of the bacterial wax coat (Fig. 47).

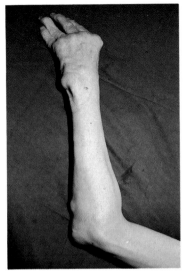

Fig. 44 Rheumatoid nodules.

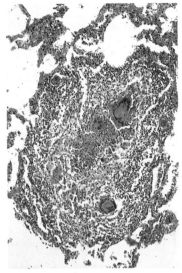

Fig. 45 Miliary tuberculous granulomas in the lung.

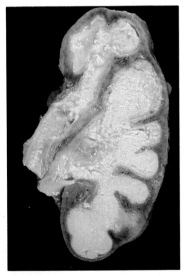

Fig. 46 Extensive caseation in the kidney.

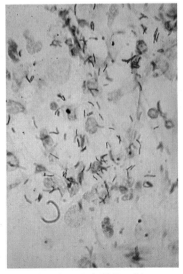

Fig. 47 *M. tuberculosis* (Z–N stain).

Gross appearance Chronic inflammation may appear as a chronic abscess (Fig. 48) or ulcer, or there may be caseous necrosis with cavity formation. Fibrosis and thickening of the wall of hollow organs, e.g. the small bowel in Crohn's disease (Fig. 49), may be marked, and may result in stenosis or stricture formation.

Microscopic appearance The histology varies with the causative agent. There are some common features.

- Active inflammation, tissue destruction and healing proceed concurrently, and fibrosis is prominent.
- The inflammatory infiltrate is mixed and includes neutrophils and eosinophils, macrophage-derived cells (epithelioid cells, giant cells), plasma cells, lymphocytes and fibroblasts. This mixture of cells is often referred to as a granulomatous reaction.

Granuloma
Granuloma is the term applied to a mass composed of granulation tissue, fibrous tissue and inflammatory cells, occasionally associated with foci of necrosis and abscesses. The use of the term has been restricted in some countries to mean a more specific collection of altered macrophages, e.g. the epithelioid cells and Langhan's giant cells found in tuberculosis (Fig. 5, p. 4) and in Crohn's disease (Fig. 50).

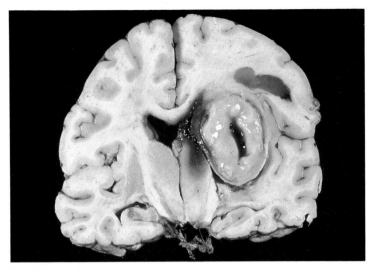

Fig. 48 Abscess in brain.

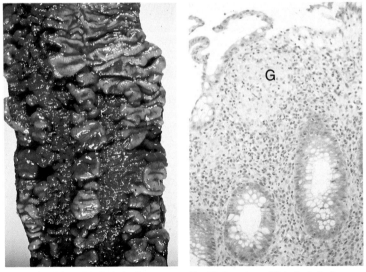

Fig. 49 Small bowel in Crohn's disease.

Fig. 50 Granuloma (G) in Crohn's disease.

9 / Healing

Control of healing This is extremely complex and poorly understood. The process of healing depends upon the continuing production of appropriate cells by resting cells re-entering the cell cycle (Fig. 51).

Contact inhibition

This occurs when cells grown in culture grow into a monolayer. A breach in the monolayer stimulates cell division and the breach is healed; cell division stops when contact is made. As cells flatten on a culture plate protein synthesis increases and cell cycle time diminishes. This may be relevant to wound healing.

Chemical mediators

These may be important in healing. Chalones are putative chemical mediators which inhibit stem cell division. Numerous polypeptide growth factors have been identified: platelet-derived growth factor (PDGF) is derived from the alpha granules and binds to vascular smooth muscle; epidermal growth factor (EGF) stimulates epidermal proliferation. Neutrophil polymorphs, macrophages, fibroblasts and nerves all produce similar factors.

Factors influencing healing
• Superimposed infection delays healing.
• Poor blood supply reduces essential nutrients; killing of phagocytosed bacteria requires additional O_2 and so polymorph function is reduced.
• Vitamin C is required for collagen synthesis; deficiency results in defective collagen, wound strength is diminished and capillary basement membrane is weakened.
• Steroid hormone treatment causes decreased polymorph and macrophage numbers, and diminished fibroblast proliferation.
• Zinc is required for collagen synthesis.

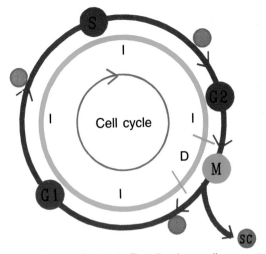

Fig. 51 Diagram of cell cycle. The cell cycle normally takes from 24 hours to several days depending on the length of the G1 phase. (M = mitosis, D = division, G1 = pre-synthetic phase, S = DNA synthetic phase, G2 = pre-mitotic phase, I = interphase and SC = stable cell.)

Skin wounds

*Primary
intention*
Surgical wounds are cleanly incised, and the edges
closely apposed by sutures to minimize the defect that
must be bridged. There are several stages.

- Blood escapes from vessels and fills the gap
  (Fig. 52A).
- Fibrin clot binds the edges together loosely and
  dries on the surface to form a scab (Fig. 52B).
- An acute inflammatory reaction develops around the
  wound in 24 hours and the fluid exudate adds more
  fibrin, polymorphs and macrophages. These release
  lytic enzymes which commence digestion of the clot.
- Epithelial regeneration from the wound edge bridges
  the gap usually within 48 hours. Within 24 hours
  of the damage a 3–4 mm zone of epithelial cells
  around the wound begin to show enlargement of
  the basal cells with flattening of the rete ridges. The
  cells slide over one another as they migrate to cover
  the defect. The cells only move over viable tissue
  and so tunnel beneath the clot forming a plane of
  cleavage between dead and viable tissue. The
  regenerated epithelium also extends around the
  suture material (Fig. 52C).

Because there is minimal tissue damage and loss
the repair of the tissue is effected with only minor
disruption to the architecture (Fig. 53).

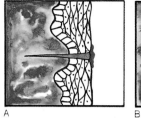
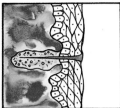

A   B

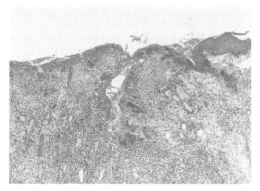

C

Fig. 52 Diagram of skin wound healing by primary intention.
A: the wound fills with small amounts of blood and a scab
forms on the surface. B: epithelium grows under the blood
clot and a little granulation tissue grows into the wound.
C: collagen bonds the wound edges and minimal scar tissue
results.

Fig. 53 Healing skin wound.

Skin wounds (contd)

Granulation tissue

In the underlying connective tissue capillaries, macrophages and fibroblasts proliferate to form granulation tissue.

- New vessels form as solid cords of cells sprouting from the existing vessels. Initially they have no basement membrane, and leak protein-rich fluid and cells. As they grow they unite with other cords and develop a lumen, re-establishing the circulation; transformation to venules and arterioles occurs in a few days.
- Fibroblasts migrate into the wound from surrounding connective tissue and produce type I and III collagen (Fig. 54). This joins the wound edges, but is of low tensile strength. Type III fibres are gradually converted into type I collagen over 6 months as it aligns along lines of stress (Fig. 55). Fibroblast proliferation may result in scarring and fibrous stricture formation, particularly in narrow tubes such as the oesophagus, ureter or urethra.
- The presence of macrophages and polymorphs attracts the fibroblasts and capillaries. Macrophages produce various growth factors including transforming growth factor (TGFβ), basic fibroblast growth factor (bFGF), interleukin 1 (Il-1) and platelet derived growth factor (PDGF) which stimulate fibroblast activation and proliferation. Angiogenesis is stimulated by tumour necrosis factor (TNFα) and bFGF. (TNF was first isolated from tumour tissue but is now known to have a wide distribution.)

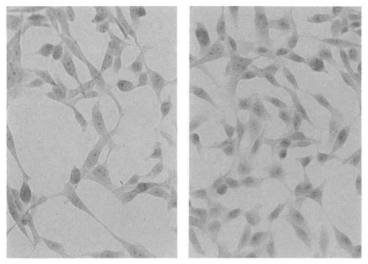

Fig. 54 Fibroblasts in tissue culture (left: immunoperoxidase stain for vimentin; right: H & E).

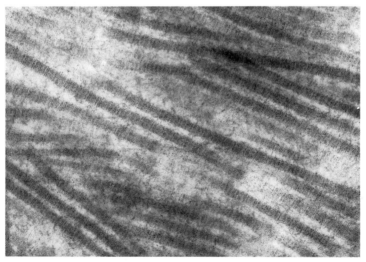

Fig. 55 Electron micrograph of collagen fibres exhibiting banding pattern.

Skin wounds (contd)

Secondary intention
In an open wound (Fig. 56) the edges are widely separated and more blood clot is formed, so larger numbers of polymorphs and macrophages are required to digest this. Epithelial regeneration takes longer, and granulation tissue is more important, forming a red granular surface in the base of the wound. The capillaries run perpendicular to the surface, accounting for the granular appearance.

The major features of this form of healing are:

- The high vascularity and inflammatory infiltrate result in a marked antibacterial activity.
- Collagen is initially laid down perpendicularly but once epithelial cover is present realignment to the horizontal occurs.
- Myofibroblasts (Fig. 57) with anchor points on both sides of the wound contract and pull the edges together, reducing the surface area for epithelial regrowth.
- In a heavily infected wound the outpouring of inflammatory cells on to the surface inhibits fibroblast proliferation and epithelial regeneration.

Various factors can influence wound healing; these can be local (infection, poor blood supply, excessive movement, foreign material and exposure to ionizing radiation) or systemic (poor nutrition, immunosuppression, renal failure, cachexia due to neoplasia). Wounds of the lower limb take longer to heal than those of the face or upper limbs because of relatively poor blood supply, particularly in the elderly with peripheral vascular disease or varicose veins. Patients who are immunosuppressed as a result of diabetes mellitus, steroid treatment, renal failure or primary haematological disorders exhibit delayed wound healing.

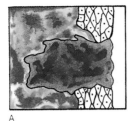
A

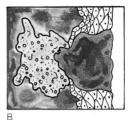
B

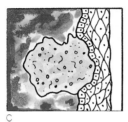
C

Fig. 56 Diagram of skin wound healing by secondary intention. A: wound fills with blood clot. B: abundant granulation tissue forms in the base of the wound and epithelium grows under the clot. C: the vascularity of the resulting bulky scar tissue gradually decreases.

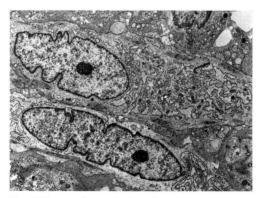

Fig. 57 Electron micrograph of myofibroblast.

10 / **Repair of fractures**

Following fracture of a bone, primary union is unusual, and secondary union is the rule. The forces required to cause a fracture result in extensive haemorrhage and displacement of the bone ends (Figs 58 & 59).

The basic healing processes are similar to those described in skin wounds, modified by the tissue reactions of bone.

Main stages
- Two cuffs of bone are laid down by the periosteum around the bone ends and these unite to form an external splint or callus, immobilizing the bone ends (Figs 58 & 59 and Figs 60 & 61, p. 44).
- Medullary cavity capillaries proliferate into the necrotic marrow, accompanied by macrophages, fibroblasts and osteoblasts.
- Osteoblasts lay down new bone, while osteoclasts remove dead bone. There may be some resorption of cortical bone resulting in widening of the fracture gap.
- The gap is closed by the production of granulation tissue.

Union
Union may occur in two ways.

Direct ossification. This is the result of osteogenic cells from the medulla and provisional callus migrating into the area and laying down bone. It may be preceded by cartilage formation, particularly if the bone ends are mobile.

Fibrous union. This results from proliferation of periosteal fibroblasts and the gap becomes heavily collagenized and then ossified. Ossification may be slow (resulting in delayed union) or may stop (resulting in non-union).

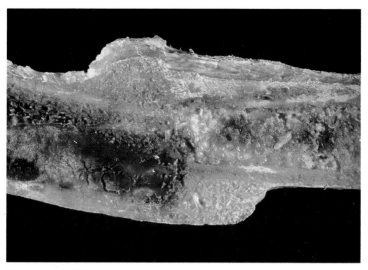
Fig. 58 Fracture of femur.

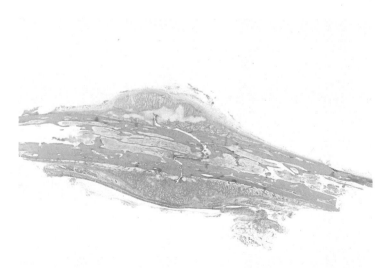
Fig. 59 Fracture of rib.

Callus Histologically, callus consists of highly cellular tissue made up of spindle cells derived from periosteal progenitor cells. This is an actively proliferating tissue which may be misinterpreted as a sarcoma. Eventually these cells develop into osteoblasts forming osteoid and bone, and chondrocytes producing cartilage (Figs 60 & 61).

Remodelling Once union has occurred and movement has been restored, the new bone is remodelled according to the imposed stresses.

- Excess external callus is removed, and woven bone is gradually replaced by stronger lamellar bone.
- Medullary callus is removed, and the medullary cavity re-established. This may take a year.

Complications These are related to the fracture itself or to part of the healing process.

Haemorrhage. This may be so severe as to require transfusion, particularly in femoral fractures.

Bone necrosis. This may occur, particularly if blood vessels are torn. The head of the femur and the scaphoid are examples.

Severe crushing. This may cause damage to medullary fat with resultant fat embolism (p. 73).

Non-union. This may occur if there is a poor blood supply, periosteal damage, bone necrosis, poor immobilization, or infection. The collagenized union may become cartilagenous and a pseudo-arthrosis or false joint forms.

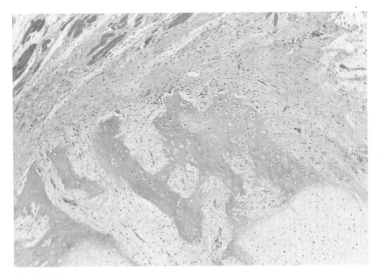

Fig. 60 Callus.

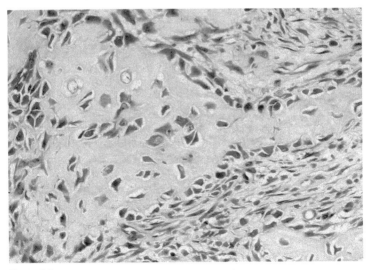

Fig. 61 Callus.

11 / **Repair of other tissues**

The healing scheme outlined for skin wounds and fractures can be applied to other tissues, for example myocardium (Fig. 62), although they may have individual differences.

Tissue types Tissues are of three main cell types:
- *Labile cells* continue to divide throughout life, e.g. skin, gastrointestinal tract, haemopoietic marrow, endometrium.
- *Stable cells* stop dividing after maturity, but retain the ability to divide, e.g. liver, renal tubular epithelium (Fig. 63), pancreas and thyroid.
- *Permanent cells* lose their ability to divide after infancy, e.g. neurones.

Repair The ability to divide obviously affects the capability of a tissue to repair itself.
- Tendons consist of dense collagenous tissue which is relatively avascular and slow to heal.
- Cartilage remains metabolically active but has a limited ability to produce collagen to repair defects.
- Peripheral nerves can regenerate. The section distal to transection degenerates (Wallerian degeneration); Schwann cells proliferate in the neurilemmal sheath to produce channels along which the axons can regenerate and this may result in re-innervation of the distal tissue if the cut ends are close together. If the ends are widely separated the axon sprouts protrude in profusion producing a traumatic neuroma (Fig. 64).

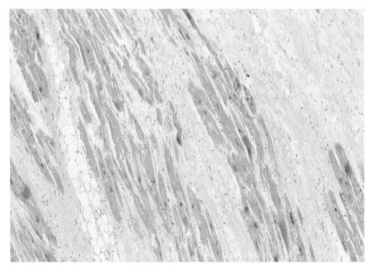

Fig. 62 Repair after a myocardial infarction.

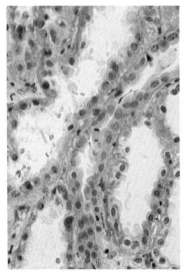

Fig. 63 Acute tubular necrosis.

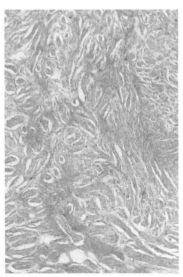

Fig. 64 Traumatic neuroma.

12 / **Organization**

Definition   The process by which the body deals with inert or dead tissue (e.g. fibrin, blood clot, necrotic tissue) is called organization.

Mechanism   Macrophages, polymorphs, young capillaries and fibroblasts are all involved, growing into the non-viable tissue, removing debris, and revascularizing it (Figs 65 & 66).

Haematomas in wounds have to be organized before healing can occur and this will delay the healing process.

Complications   While this is a physiological process which should return the tissue to normality—resolution—this ideal state of affairs is achieved only rarely. In the pleural and pericardial cavities (Fig. 67) fibrinous exudates may be organized with resultant obliteration of the potential space and replacement of the exudate by fibrous tissue giving restricted movement of the lungs or heart. Healing by fibrosis also occurs where there is the removal of substantial amounts of dead or dying tissue, the resultant scar marking the site of previous injury. For example an area of dense white fibrous tissue may remain in the left ventricle at the site of a previous myocardial infarction. Contraction of scar tissue in superficial sites may give rise to disfiguring cosmetic results and loss of function, e.g. around a joint.

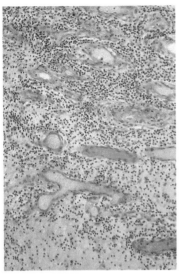

Fig. 65 Granulation tissue.

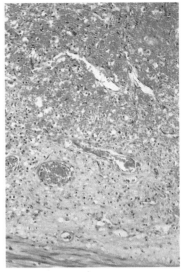

Fig. 66 Organization of thrombus in a vein.

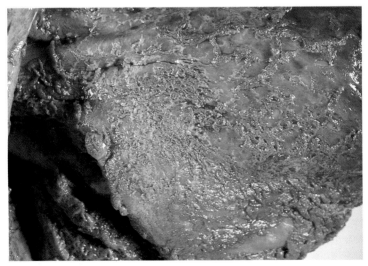

Fig. 67 Pericarditis.

13 / Hypertrophy and hyperplasia

Definitions   **Hyperplasia** is an increase in the numbers of parenchymal cells as a result of increased demand.

Hypertrophy is an increase in the size of the cells (Fig. 68).

Hypertrophy and hyperplasia may occur together, although their relative importance may vary.

Aetiology   There are two main causes:
- *Increased functional demand* particularly affects muscular organs, e.g. left ventricular hypertrophy in systemic hypertension (Fig. 69), skeletal muscle fibres increase in size in athletes, bladder muscle hypertrophies as a result of outflow obstruction caused by prostatic hypertrophy.
- *Excessive hormonal stimulation* may affect a specific target organ, e.g. in pregnancy placental and corpus luteal hormones stimulate an increase in the number and size of breast lobules prior to lactation (Fig. 70). More generalized effects result from overproduction of growth hormone by the pituitary resulting in gigantism if it occurs in childhood or adolescence before the epiphyses have fused, or in acromegaly in the adult.

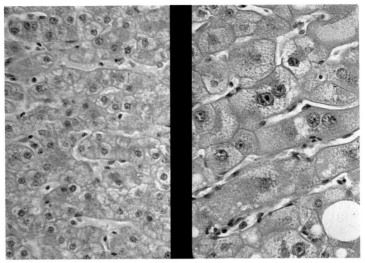

Fig. 68 Hypertrophy of hepatocytes (right) with normal liver for comparison (left).

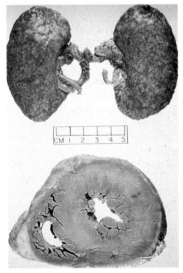

Fig. 69 Left ventricular hypertrophy in patient with malignant hypertension.

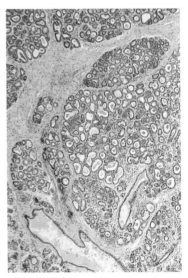

Fig. 70 Hypertrophy of breast tissue in pregnancy.

14 / Water and salt loss

Water comprises 60% of the body: 40 litres is intracellular, 10 litres extracellular. Since the latter contains most of the sodium, restricted water intake results in the extracellular compartment becoming hypertonic and water is withdrawn from the cells. In salt depletion the extracellular fluid becomes hypotonic, water is excreted and the extracellular volume decreases. Water administration results in further dilution and more diffusion of water into cells.

Dehydration

Insufficient intake of water results in a series of changes:
- reduction in urine volume, and rise in specific gravity
- the renin–angiotensin–aldosterone system stimulates active sodium retention and potassium excretion (Fig. 71)
- plasma sodium, chloride and urea rise.

In fatal cases the total body water may be severely reduced and death is the result of increased intracellular osmotic pressure.

Salt depletion

This is a commoner cause of serious effects than simple water loss, and is also more likely to go unnoticed clinically.

Aetiology
- Excessive sweating (particularly if treated solely by water replacement) results in salt loss.
- Vomiting and diarrhoea cause salt and water depletion and cause alkalosis and acidosis respectively.
- Potassium may be lost preferentially, e.g. from large villous adenomas of the rectum (Fig. 157, p. 112) with consequential severe vacuolation of renal tubules (Fig. 72).

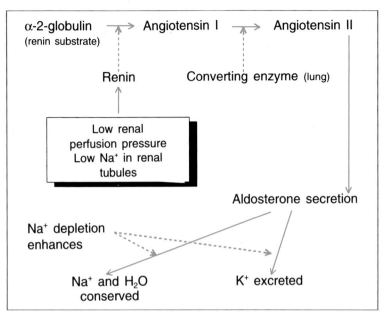

Fig. 71 Diagram of the renin–angiotensin–aldosterone system.

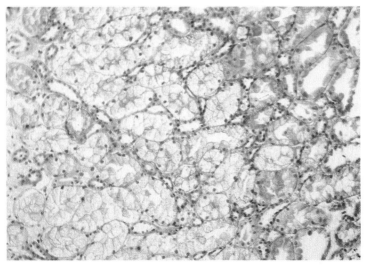

Fig. 72 Renal tubules in potassium deficiency.

15 / **Oedema**

Definition   Oedema is an abnormal increase in the amount of interstitial fluid and may be localized or generalized.

Localized oedema

Aetiology   Local oedema is caused by:

- Increased net loss of fluid into the interstitial tissue (Fig. 73). This occurs typically in acute inflammation in which increased blood flow and vascular permeability with increased interstitial plasma protein results in increased osmotic pressure. Lymphatic drainage is increased but does not keep pace with the increased flow. Venous drainage may be reduced diminishing the movement of fluid from the interstitial to the vascular compartment. This form of oedema is characterized by 'pitting' on pressure (Fig. 74).
- Failure to remove fluid from the interstitial tissue as a result of lymphatic blockage. This occurs as a result of lymphatic invasion and obstruction by tumour, or secondary to surgery or radiotherapy. The interstitial fluid is rich in plasma proteins which stimulate production of connective tissue. This form does not 'pit' on pressure. Lymphoedema of the arm following breast cancer surgery and radiotherapy to the axilla is the commonest example.

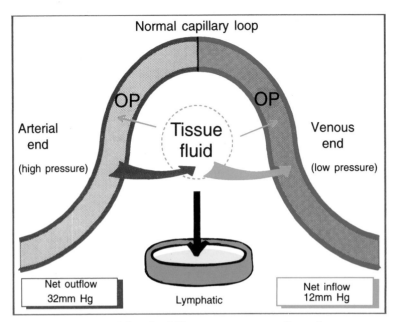

Fig. 73 Diagram of factors influencing fluid movement across a capillary wall.

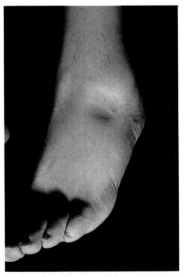

Fig. 74 'Pitting' oedema of foot.

Generalized oedema

Generalized oedema tends to accumulate in serous cavities (ascites and hydrothorax). In the skin the localized fluid may be temporarily displaced by pressure ('pitting' oedema) (Fig. 74, p. 54).

This indicates an attempt to regulate an increase in the intravascular volume by redistributing fluid to the interstitial tissues. In the adult an increase in body weight of 5 kg precedes the appearance of oedema.

Aetiology There are several causes:

Cardiac oedema. This occurs in heart failure. If the right heart fails there is venous congestion, affecting initially the dependent areas, then the serous cavities. In left heart failure the venous congestion affects the lungs, giving pulmonary oedema.

Renal oedema. This results from various diseases. In acute post-infectious glomerulonephritis there may be hypertension, generalized oedema and oliguria (the *nephritic syndrome*). In membranous glomerulonephritis (Figs 75 & 76) there may be severe proteinuria, generalized oedema and raised blood lipids (the *nephrotic syndrome*). The loss of albumin which usually maintains plasma osmotic pressure results in increasing oedema and decreased plasma volume with activation of the renin–angiotensin–aldosterone system.

Nutritional oedema. This is seen in severe malnutrition and reflects a dramatic fall in plasma protein. Other factors involved in its development include:

• vitamin B deficiency
• loss of fat.

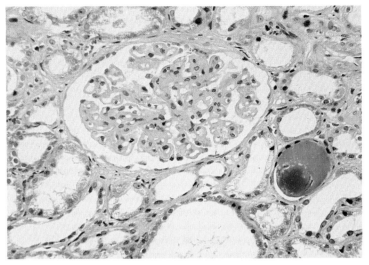

Fig. 75 Membranous glomerulonephritis (Masson stain).

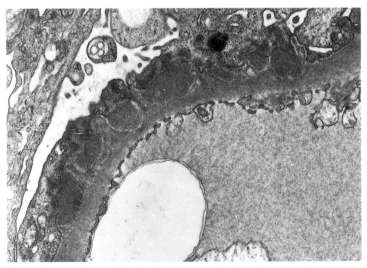

Fig. 76 Electron micrograph showing immune complex deposition in membranous glomerulonephritis.

16 / Shock

Definition   Shock is the series of changes which occur after a severe and sudden drop in cardiac output. These changes are an attempt to maintain an adequate blood supply to essential organs often at the expense of other tissues, which become ischaemic (Fig. 77).

Clinical types   **Hypovolaemic shock.** This occurs following severe haemorrhage (Fig. 78) or secondary to loss of other fluids, e.g. exudation of plasma accompanying extensive burns.

Cardiogenic shock. This arises as a result of a sudden and profound drop in cardiac output secondary to myocardial infarction, rupture of a valve cusp, major arrhythmia or cardiac tamponade.

Septic shock. This develops in patients with septicaemia or severe localized infections. The aetiology is not completely understood, but it is usually associated with Gram-negative infections (e.g. *Esch. coli*, *Proteus* spp, *Klebsiella*). When these organisms die they release endotoxins which are believed to cause the features of 'endotoxic' shock. Patients dying from this develop multi-organ failure including severe respiratory distress (Fig. 79) secondary to fibrin deposition in the lung alveoli.

Pathogenesis   Gram-negative endotoxins activate Hageman factor and hence initiate these systems:

- complement
- coagulation
- fibrinolytic
- kinin.

Platelets are also activated.

Occasional cases of septic shock are associated with Gram-positive infections. Exotoxins have been implicated in the aetiology of these cases.

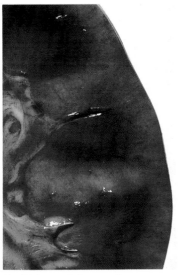

Fig. 77 Acute tubular necrosis.

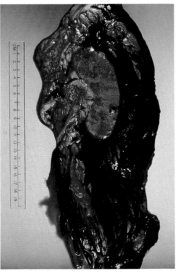

Fig. 78 Perinephric haematoma following renal biopsy.

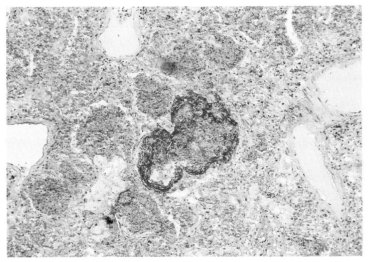

Fig. 79 'Shock' lung (MSB stain).

17 / Changes in total blood flow

Increase in total blood flow

An increase in total blood flow may be due to:
- Generalized arteriolar smooth muscle relaxation. This may be physiological as in the effects of strenuous exercise or can be pathological.
- An increase in cardiac output to compensate for tissue hypoxia. In hypoxia there is a decrease in the total amount of O_2 delivered to the tissues; e.g. in anaemia (Fig. 80) or in patients with deficient lung function.
- An increased metabolic rate, e.g. in patients with thyrotoxicosis, or who have a fever secondary to an infection such as an acute appendicitis (Fig. 81).
- A marked local increase in vascularity in, for example, Paget's disease of bone (Fig. 82), an arteriovenous fistula or an extensive inflammatory condition of the skin may result in increased cardiac output.

Reduction in total blood flow

Sudden reduction in total blood flow results in the syndrome of shock (p. 57).

In chronic heart failure output does not meet with the tissue demands for O_2, etc. The main causes of such failure are ischaemic heart disease, heart valve defects and hypertension.

In underactivity of the thyroid gland there is a decrease in total blood flow, but this is compensated for by decrease in the tissue requirements for nutrients due to the lowered metabolic rate.

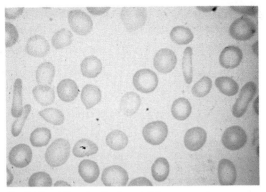

Fig. 80 Blood film showing iron deficiency anaemia.

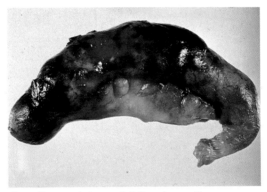

Fig. 81 Hyperaemia in acutely inflamed appendix.

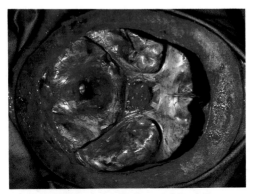

Fig. 82 Hyperaemia in Paget's disease of the skull.

18 / Local reduction in blood flow

Clinical types **Ischaemia**. This is a deficiency, either relative or absolute, in the supply of blood; it is often associated with total or partial obstruction of an artery (Figs 83 & 84). In the presence of a collateral circulation sudden blockage of one vessel results in the dilatation of the others. In the elderly the presence of disease in the collateral vessels (atheroma, etc.) prevents their efficient dilatation and blockage of one vessel may result in death of tissue despite the apparent presence of an alternative circulation. The most serious result of ischaemia is infarction.

Infarction. This is tissue necrosis resulting from a reduction or loss of blood supply, the dead tissue being referred to as an infarct.

Pathogenesis Infarction is usually caused by obstruction of one or more arteries by *thrombosis* or *embolism*.

The size of an infarct depends on:
- the size of the vessel blocked
- the extent of the blockage
- whether the blockage was sudden or gradual
- the availability of collateral vessels
- the susceptibility of the tissue to ischaemia.

Gross appearance The appearance of the infarct depends on the tissue involved: heart, kidney and spleen show a coagulative pattern (p. 3) while necrotic brain tissue is colliquative (p. 3). Lung infarcts are wedge-shaped and haemorrhagic because of their dual blood supply. Bowel infarcts may be secondary to blockage of a mesenteric vessel by thrombus, or secondary to the blood supply being compromised by twisting of a loop of bowel (*volvulus*) or by a loop being impacted in a hernial sac. Bowel infarcts tend to be haemorrhagic and are rapidly infected by the bowel flora (*gangrene*) (Fig. 85).

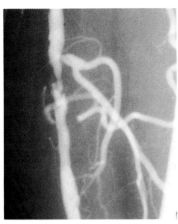

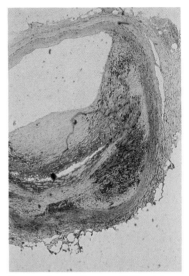

Fig. 83 Stenosis of femoral artery with collateral vessels (X-ray after contrast injection).

Fig. 84 Atheroma in artery (lipid stain).

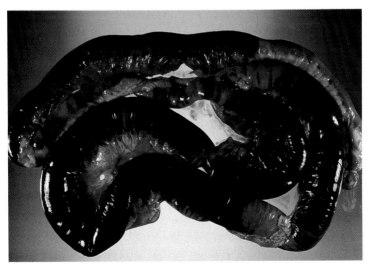

Fig. 85 Small bowel infarction.

19 / Haemostasis and thrombosis

Blood is fluid within the vascular tree but if blood vessels are damaged, an elaborate protective mechanism is activated to secure local haemostasis; a solid adherent mass of material forms (a *thrombus*) to prevent blood loss.

Definition   Thrombosis is the formation of a solid or semisolid mass from the constituents of the blood within the vascular system and during life (Fig. 86 and Fig. 87, p. 66).

Thrombi formed in fast flowing blood consist mainly of aggregated platelets and entrapped fibrin. They enlarge slowly and are pale because of the low content of red blood cells (RBCs).

A thrombus formed in a stagnant column of blood is similar to blood which clotted in a glass tube: soft, gelatinous and red, and composed of an extensive fibrin meshwork in which are trapped large numbers of RBCs (Fig. 88, p. 66).

Aetiology   The following predispose to thrombosis:
- abnormalities in the flow of blood
- abnormalities in the composition of the blood
- abnormalities in the heart or blood vessels containing the blood.

Fibrinolysis
The coagulation cascade is constantly being invoked to deal with the innumerable small defects which occur within the vascular system. Such a repair system also requires a removal system to dispose of the coagulum once it has fulfilled its function. The fibrinolytic system of enzymes (Fig. 89, p. 66) subserves this purpose. In the normal individual, the coagulation and fibrinolytic systems are finely balanced. If this balance is upset then, at one extreme, there may be disseminated intravascular coagulation, whilst at the other, inappropriate fibrinolytic activity may cause haemorrhage.

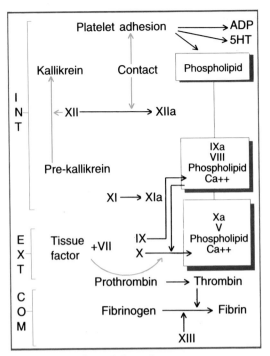

Fig. 86 Diagram of coagulation pathway.

Repair of vascular injury

Endothelium plays a prominent role in many pathological processes, synthesizing numerous regulatory molecules. These include factors stimulating or inhibiting coagulation and platelets, promoting or inhibiting fibrinolysis, and altering blood flow:

Activation	Inhibition
Coagulation factors III, V and VIII	Heparin, thrombomodulin
Platelet activating factor	Prostacyclin
Tissue plasminogen activator	Plasminogen activator inhibitor
Angiotensin converting enzyme	Endothelium-derived relaxing factor (EDRF) (nitric oxide)

In response to injury endothelial cells may retract exposing underlying connective tissues. These tissues, including collagen, laminin and fibronectin, promote platelet adhesion and activation and provide a surface which stimulates the intrinsic coagulation pathway. The endothelial cells play a balancing role between the opposing forces of haemorrhage and thrombosis. Minor endothelial damage in small blood vessels is a frequent occurrence and is repaired by the adherence of aggregated platelets to the damaged section followed by the growth of endothelium over the platelets to restore continuity of the vessel lining.

In more severe injury, temporary vasoconstriction restricts the immediate blood loss; platelets then adhere to the torn collagen fibres at the edge of the wound and, together with fibrin strands, form a solid mass of tissue (*haemostatic plug*) which prevents further bleeding. The plug is covered by endothelial growth, restoring the continuity of the vessel lining and is finally removed by organization.

Patients who are thrombocytopenic (deficient in platelets) may show spontaneous haemorrhages from small blood vessels whilst patients with coagulation defects, such as haemophiliacs, may present with bleeding problems, e.g. spontaneous joint haemorrhage.

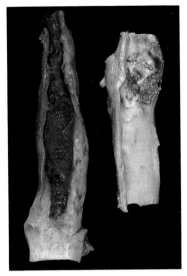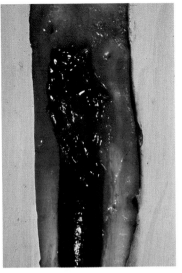

Fig. 87 Thrombus in carotid artery.

Fig. 88 Post-mortem clot in femoral artery.

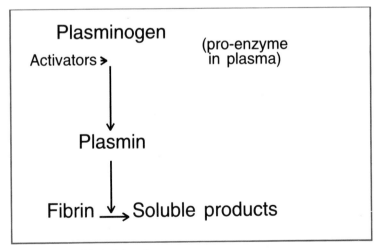

Fig. 89 Diagram of fibrinolytic pathway.

Sites of thrombus formation

Heart. The most common thrombi found in the ventricles are areas of mural thrombus overlying sites of myocardial infarction (Fig. 90). The flat red/brown thrombus is formed in relation to the disturbed blood flow over the akinetic segment and also to the diffusion of tissue breakdown products (factor III) from the damaged muscle.

Thrombi may also be found on the valve cusps in certain diseases and are referred to as vegetations (Fig. 91). In rheumatic fever the valve cusps are damaged along the line of apposition and tiny pink/grey vegetations along this line represent the laying down of platelets and fibrin. In subacute bacterial endocarditis the valve cusps are colonized by microorganisms and large crumbling vegetations of mixed thrombus are formed.

Arteries. Blood flow in the arteries is rapid and hence thrombosis is unlikely unless there is some predisposing disease of the vessel wall, e.g. atheroma.

In the smaller arteries, e.g. the coronary and cerebral vessels, this mural thrombus may cause occlusion. In the aorta, atheroma causes weakening of the wall and eventually gives rise to localized areas of dilatation (*aneurysms*) (Fig. 92) causing disturbed blood flow along the vessel with the formation of laminated thrombus.

Traumatic injury to the wall of an artery is an obvious cause of thrombosis.

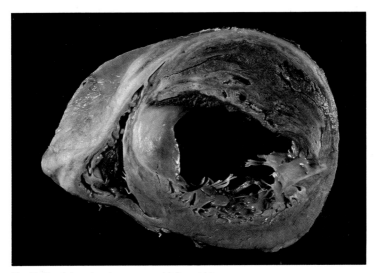

Fig. 90 Mural thrombus in aneurysmal left ventricle.

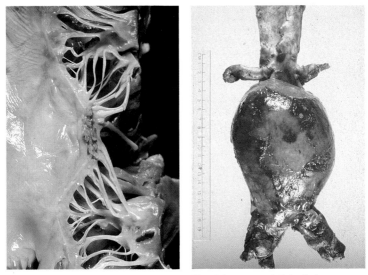

Fig. 91 Vegetations on mitral valve cusps.   **Fig. 92** Aneurysm of abdominal aorta.

Sites of thrombus formation (contd)

Veins. Thrombus in the veins of the lower limbs (Fig. 93) is common in patients who are:
• bedridden
• recovering from major surgery or trauma
• pregnant or postpartum.

Post-surgery or post-trauma patients show increased numbers of platelets with increased adhesiveness while pregnant patients show a decreased venous return from the lower limbs due to the pressure of the enlarged uterus on the pelvic veins.

Local infections may give rise to inflammation of the veins (*phlebitis*) and secondary thrombosis; this may also be seen affecting multiple veins (*migrating thrombophlebitis*) in some patients with visceral malignancy, e.g. cancer of the pancreas. Leukaemia and polycythaemia rubra vera also have an increased liability to venous thrombosis due to increased viscosity.

Capillaries. Thrombosis in capillary networks is found in acute inflammatory reactions, in the Arthus reaction secondary to endothelial damage and in disseminated intravascular coagulation (DIC) (Fig. 94).

Sequelae

Organization of thrombi occurs in the same way as other digestible tissue. In veins the shrinkage of the soft red thrombus gives rise to fluid-filled spaces which become endothelialized and which, together with new vessels growing in from the wall, may link up to form channels, eventually restoring a lumen (Fig. 95). In arteries the denser thrombi are less readily digested and recanalization occurs much less frequently.

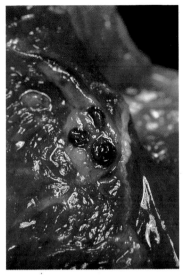

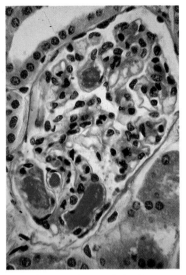

Fig. 93 Deep calf vein thrombosis.

Fig. 94 Intravascular coagulation in glomerular capillaries.

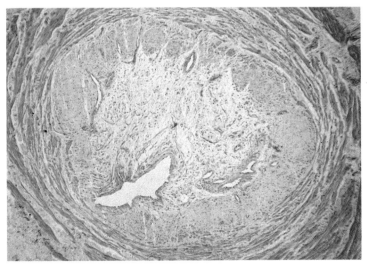

Fig. 95 Recanalization of thrombus in vein.

20 / **Embolism**

Definition Embolism is the transfer of abnormal material by means of the bloodstream and its impaction in a vessel.

Clinical types Emboli may consist of:
- a fragment of thrombus
- a portion of ulcerating atheromatous plaque (Figs 96 & 97)
- tumour cells
- bone marrow (fat) (Fig. 98)
- air or nitrogen bubbles
- amniotic fluid
- foreign material
- septic tissue.

The site at which the embolus lodges depends on its site of origin; e.g. emboli originating in the left side of the heart or arteries will be found in the systemic circulation whilst those originating in the venous system will be found in the pulmonary arterial circulation. In patients with a patent foramen ovale, emboli from the venous system can pass from the right to the left side of the heart and hence end up in the systemic circulation (*paradoxical embolism*).

Sequelae Emboli to the systemic circulation block the blood supply to the appropriate tissue.

Systemic arterial embolism. This usually occurs in patients with severe atheroma of the lower aorta, and results in embolization of the femoral vessels with acute ischaemia of the affected lower limb. Unless the circulation is rapidly re-established by embolectomy or the use of streptokinase infusion peripheral gangrene will develop with the need for amputation.

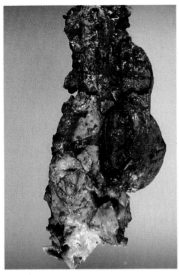

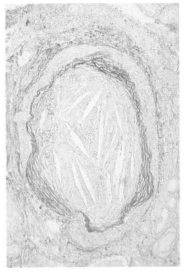

Fig. 96 Atheroma of aorta.

Fig. 97 Atheromatous embolism in kidney.

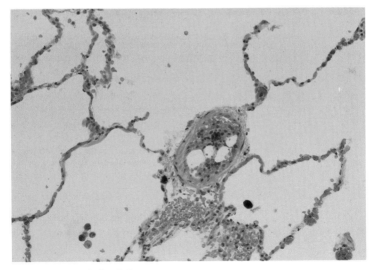

Fig. 98 Marrow embolism in lung.

Sequelae
(contd)

Pulmonary emboli. Emboli originating in the deep calf veins have effects which depend on the size of the embolism and hence the extent to which the pulmonary arterial flow is compromised. Their effect also depends on the state of the pulmonary circulation. Massive pulmonary embolism (Fig. 99) (>95% blockage of the pulmonary arterial outflow) causes instant death whilst lesser but serious degrees of blockage (>50%) gives rise to acute right-heart failure. Blockage of a moderate- or small-sized pulmonary artery may give rise to a wedge-shaped haemorrhagic pulmonary infarct (Figs 100 & 101) with overlying pleurisy. Multiple small emboli can eventually cause pulmonary hypertension.

Septic emboli. These contain pyogenic bacteria and are now rare due to the use of antibiotics. They usually originate from foci of bacterial endocarditis or from a vein involved in suppuration. The wall of the vessel at which the embolus impacts is weakened and may dilate (*mycotic aneurysm*).

Fat emboli. These are common after the fracture of long bones and most are arrested in the pulmonary circulation (Fig. 98, p. 72). The majority are symptomless.

In major bony injury the fat embolus syndrome may occur in which fat globules may appear in the systemic circulation. The patient is confused and may show fever, breathlessness, a petechial rash and tachycardia. Oil globules may appear in the urine (Fig. 102). In severe cases there is cyanosis, haemoptysis, coma and death.

Air embolism. This occurs when negative pressure in the neck veins sucks air into a defect in the vein walls. Small volumes cause no problems, being rapidly absorbed; 100 ml can cause acute distress and 300 ml can prove fatal.

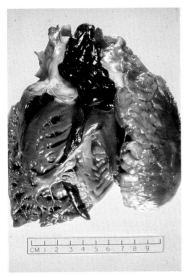

Fig. 99 Thrombus in pulmonary outflow from heart.

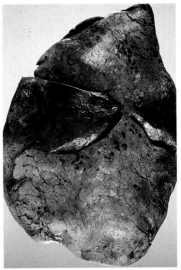

Fig. 100 Pulmonary embolism and infarction.

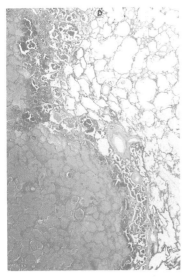

Fig. 101 Pulmonary infarction.

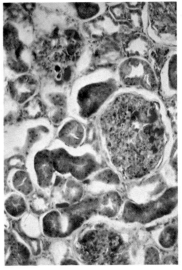

Fig. 102 Fat embolism in kidney (Oil red O stain).

21 / Amyloid

Definition Amyloid is an extracellular, fibrillar protein with a characteristic β-pleated pattern on X-ray diffraction, which is deposited in tissues in a variety of conditions.

Gross appearance Affected tissues are enlarged and appear waxy (Fig. 103). Grossly, amyloid produces a dark brown colour with Lugol's iodine (Fig. 104).

Microscopic appearance In conventional haematoxylin and eosin stained sections, amyloid is pale pink (Fig. 105). Sirius or Congo red stains give an apple green birefringence in histological sections in polarized light (Fig. 106, p. 78). Ultrastructurally, it is composed of 7.5 nm filaments which may be twisted together in pairs (Fig. 107, p. 78).

Sequelae Amyloid is found in the basement membranes of small blood vessels. In large amounts it may weaken capillaries causing petechial haemorrhages in the skin. The transfer of nutrients, salts and water across basement membranes is disrupted, the consequences depending on the organ involved.

Deposits
In most organs there is a uniform deposition of amyloid. The spleen is unusual in that while it may show uniform involvement there may also be selective white pulp deposition (*sago spleen*; Fig. 104). If renal involvement is severe, chronic renal failure supervenes. In the gastrointestinal tract atrophy of the mucosa results in diarrhoea. Cardiac involvement may present with heart failure.

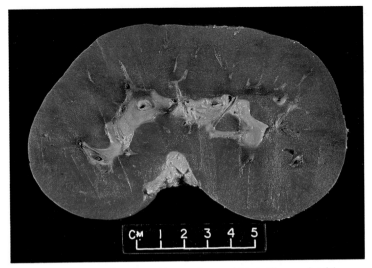

Fig. 103 Enlarged kidney in patient with secondary amyloidosis (Congo red stain).

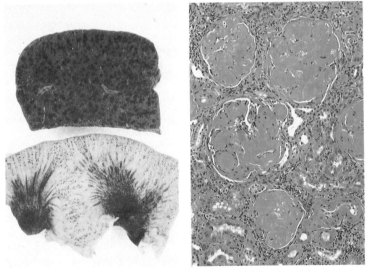

Fig. 104 'Sago' spleen and amyloid kidney (Lugol's iodine stain).

Fig. 105 Amyloid in glomeruli.

Classification Amyloid can be classified according to:
- Whether it is hereditary or acquired. There are several familial forms, e.g. familial Mediterranean fever.
- Whether it is localized or diffuse. It may rarely be confined to one organ.
- The chemical make-up of the amyloid. There are two main types: AA and AL (Fig. 108). There are other types which occur less commonly, for example transthyretin and beta-2-microglobulin amyloid and those associated with endocrine tumours (AE) and with senility (AS).

AA. The AA type of amyloid is derived from the plasma proteins, its exact origin being uncertain. It is usually secondary to:
- Chronic inflammatory diseases, e.g. TB, leprosy, syphilis, osteomyelitis, bronchiectasis and rheumatoid arthritis.
- Hodgkin's disease.
- Miscellaneous ailments including Crohn's disease and SLE. The amyloid is deposited in the liver, kidney and spleen and death due to amyloid is as a result of renal failure.

AL. The AL type of amyloid is derived from the N-terminal portion of immunoglobulin light chains. It is deposited in the heart, gastrointestinal tract and skin, and death is secondary to heart failure.
Secondary light chain amyloid can occur in patients with multiple myeloma, a tumour of plasma cells with excessive immunoglobulin production.

AE. Characteristically this is found in medullary carcinoma of the thyroid where it is formed from fragments of precalcitonin.

AS. There are two types:
- ASb—amyloid senile cerebrovascular deposits—seen in patients with Alzheimer's disease.
- ASc—senile amyloidosis—fibrils derived from atrial natriuretic peptide.

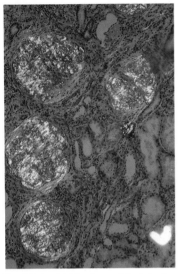

Fig. 106 Amyloid in glomeruli (polarized light birefringence with Congo red stain).

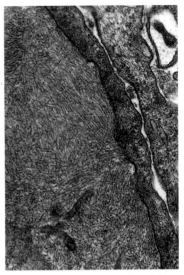

Fig. 107 Electron micrograph of amyloid fibrils.

Amyloid				
Type	Structure	Aetiology	Site of deposition	Derivation
AA	β-Pleated sheets	Secondary to chronic suppuration	Liver, spleen and kidney	Polypeptide formed from SAA protein
AL	β-Pleated sheets	Primary in the elderly Secondary, in multiple myeloma	Heart, gastro-intestinal tract, skin, and muscle	Polypeptide formed from light chains IgG

Fig. 108 Table of amyloid characteristics.

22 / Hyaline and fibrinoid change

Hyaline

Definition Hyaline describes intra- or extracellular material, with a homogeneous, eosinophilic and refractile appearance under light microscopy. The term is purely descriptive and hyalin is not a distinct chemical entity.

Sites Hyaline material can be found in various sites:

- In the walls of blood vessels which are aged or have been subjected to excess pressure as in hypertension (*hyaline degeneration*) (Fig. 109).
- In the collagen and ground substance of dense fibrous tissue.
- In diabetes mellitus similar changes occur in vessel walls secondary to leakage of blood products into the vessel wall (*plasmatic vasculosis*).
- In proteinuria hyaline droplets of protein ingested by cells, may be seen in the cytoplasm of renal tubular cells. Tubular protein may also coagulate within the lumen forming hyaline protein casts (Fig. 110).
- In liver parenchymal cells, in a variety of diseases, intermediate filament protein may aggregate in the cytoplasm as Mallory's hyalin (Fig. 111).

Fibrinoid change

Definition Fibrinoid change occurs when tissues are impregnated with a hyaline material, which has the tinctorial properties of fibrin: its exact chemical constitution is still unresolved.

Sites
- In severe exudative acute inflammatory reactions, cell death may occur (*fibrinoid necrosis*). This is found in hypersensitivity states such as the Arthus reaction.
- In the base of peptic ulcers.
- In some infarcts.
- In the vascular damage of malignant hypertension (Fig. 112).
- In rheumatoid nodules.

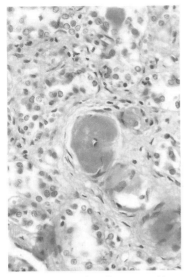

Fig. 109 Stenosis of small artery resulting from extensive hyaline change.

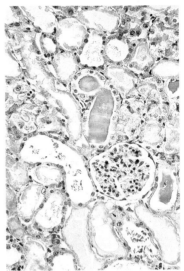

Fig. 110 Hyaline protein casts in renal tubules.

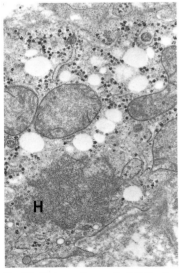

Fig. 111 Electron micrograph of Mallory's alcoholic hyalin (H) in liver.

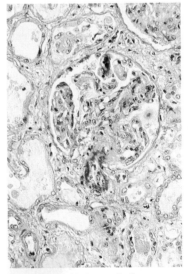

Fig. 112 Fibrinoid change of afferent glomerular arteriole in malignant hypertension (Mallory's stain).

23 / **Mucins and myxomatous change**

Definition   Mucins are mixtures of glycoproteins, which are rich in hexose polymers, and mucoproteins. They are secreted by some glandular surfaces and also by some connective tissue cells such as the chondroblast, osteoblast and the fibroblast.

Epithelial mucin
Epithelial mucin production disorders are relatively rare.

Aetiology   • Cystic fibrosis, inherited as an autosomal recessive trait, is characterized by the secretion of thick and tenacious mucin. This causes obstruction of the ducts of small mucin-secreting glands in the pancreas, bowel, bronchi (Fig. 113), biliary tree and sweat glands with glandular atrophy and loss of function. The loss of pancreatic proteolytic enzymes gives rise to malabsorption.
   • Chronic irritation of a glandular surface can lead to overproduction of mucus; in chronic bronchitis pollutants in the atmosphere cause an increase in the number and activity of the mucin glands with the production of abundant mucoid sputum (Fig. 114).
   • Some epithelial tumours are characterized by mucin production (Figs 115 & 116).

Connective tissue mucins

These are important in the ground substance of fibrous tissue, cartilage and bone. They are usually in a gel state but may be depolymerized to a fluid phase in some acute inflammatory reactions.

Clinical features   Abundant connective tissue mucin gives rise to a so-called myxomatous or myxoid appearance which can be found in a number of conditions:
   • in *Marfan's syndrome* in which a myxoid change in the media of the aorta leads to weakening and to dissecting aneurysm formation
   • in *hypothyroidism* the connective tissue changes are responsible for the characteristic facies and for the laryngeal changes which give rise to the typical hoarse voice.

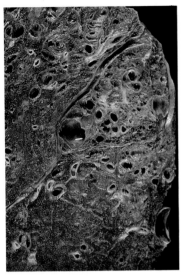

Fig. 113 Bronchiectasis from a case of cystic fibrosis.

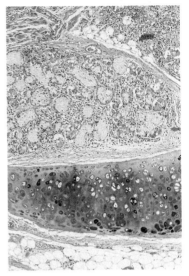

Fig. 114 Chronic bronchitis.

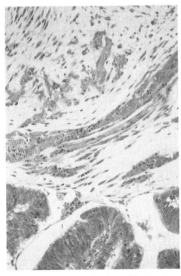

Fig. 115 Carcinoma of colon with abundant extracellular mucin.

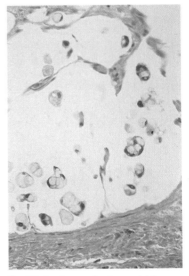

Fig. 116 Carcinoma of colon containing abundant intracellular mucin ('signet-ring' cell).

24 / Pigmentary disorders

Melanin

Definition Melanin is a sulphur-containing, iron-free pigment which varies in colour from yellow to dark brown. Formed from colourless precursors called melanogens within cells, it is manufactured in specific organelles called premelanosomes (Fig. 117). Found particularly in the melanocytes in the skin, melanin is then taken up by adjacent epidermal cells and by macrophages within the dermis.

Disorders There are a number of pathological conditions in which the amount of melanin pigment may be altered.

- In *Addison's disease* adrenal failure causes an increase in the amount of corticotrophin and β-lipotrophin released from the pituitary. These trophic hormones stimulate a general increase in melanin pigmentation in the skin.
- In *chloasma*, a condition associated with pregnancy, with ovarian disease or with the taking of oral contraceptive hormone preparations, pigmented patches appear on the face and the nipples often darken.
- Patchy depigmentation of the skin is called *vitiligo* or *leukoderma*. In the affected areas the dendritic cells lose their capacity to form pigment and are abnormal in structure.
- Excess pigment may also be associated with the presence of multiple polyps in the small bowel; a familial condition known as *Peutz–Jeghers syndrome*.
- Pigmented tumours are obviously of great importance. These may be benign (*pigmented naevi*; Fig. 118) or malignant (*melanocarcinoma*) which can be situated in the skin (Fig. 119) or in the pigmented coats of the eye (Fig. 120) (see p. 121).

However, melanosis coli is a misnomer. The excess pigmentation found in the colon is associated with the abuse of anthracene-based purgatives and is due to an excess of lipofuscin-like pigment (p. 87).

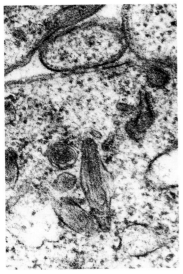

Fig. 117 Electron micrograph of premelanosomes.

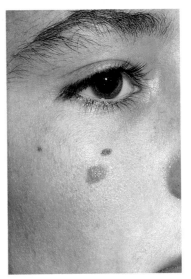

Fig. 118 Pigmented naevus.

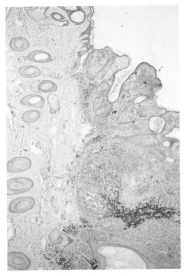

Fig. 119 Nodular melanocarcinoma.

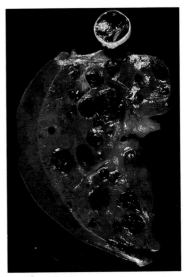

Fig. 120 Melanocarcinoma of retina with secondary deposits in the liver.

Haemoglobin

Aetiology   Pigmentation due to haemoglobin may be due to either of its main breakdown products (Fig. 121).

Biliverdin/bilirubin group. These iron-free pigments may be seen either as a local or as a generalized phenomenon. After local trauma with bleeding into the tissues, a bruise is the manifestation of the liberated pigments. Bilirubin accumulates in the bloodstream either because of increased production (e.g. in the haemolytic anaemias) or due to the failure of the liver to excrete bilirubin (e.g. due to obstruction of the common bile duct). Both entities present as jaundice.

Ferritin/haemosiderin group. Most of the iron in the body is present within the red blood cells; in the plasma iron is carried bound to a β-globulin called transferrin. Red cells are broken down by the reticulo-endothelial system, and the iron compounds are seen as haemosiderin granules in the macrophages (Fig. 122).

More widespread deposition of haemosiderin granules occurs in haemosiderosis and haemochromatosis (Fig. 123).

Disorders of iron pigmentation   ***Haemosiderosis***. This occurs in patients with excessive blood destruction as a result of chronic haemolytic anaemia or pernicious anaemia; or in patients who have had multiple blood transfusions for aplastic anaemia, in whom haemosiderin is deposited in the liver, kidney and bone marrow. It may also be found where there has been extensive and repeated tissue haemorrhage, or after dietary overload.

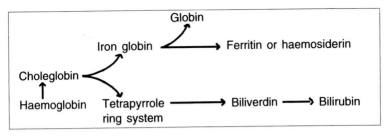

Fig. 121 Diagram of haemoglobin breakdown.

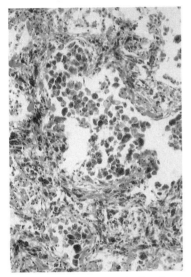

Fig. 122 Chronic venous congestion of lung.

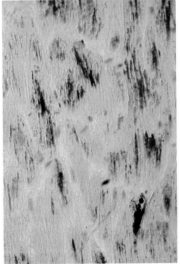

Fig. 123 Iron overload. Haemosiderin in heart muscle (Prussian blue reaction).

Disorders of iron pigmentation (contd)

Haemochromatosis. This is an inherited disease in which there is widespread tissue deposition of haemosiderin with no obvious pre-existing disease. There is an increased intake of iron from the gastrointestinal tract, although the dietary intake is normal. More common in men than women, increased absorption starts from birth and iron stores can reach levels of 20 g. Plasma transferrin levels are normal although the degree of saturation with iron may be increased. The excess iron is stored in the liver, pancreas, myocardium and skin. The iron is toxic to the tissues and patients suffer from cirrhosis (Fig. 124), diabetes, heart failure (Fig. 123, p. 86) and skin pigmentation (*bronzed diabetes*).

Malarial pigment. Haematin is a dark brown pigment produced by the malarial parasites within erythrocytes. When the adult parasite divides, the red cells are lysed and the pigment is liberated into the circulation to be ingested by macrophages in the spleen, liver and bone marrow.

Lipofuscin

Pathogenesis

This pigment represents residual breakdown products of cell metabolism found in secondary lysosomes (Fig. 125), and can be thought of as a 'wear and tear' pigment.

Microscopic appearance

As cells age finely divided yellow/brown pigment accumulates in the cytoplasm, often around the nucleus.

Gross appearance

Lipofuscin is found in wasting diseases and in atrophic tissues, particularly in smooth muscle and in heart muscle, where it gives rise to the appearance of 'brown atrophy' (Fig. 21).

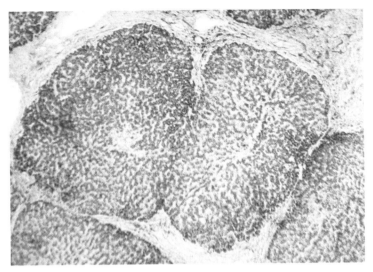

Fig. 124 Haemochromatosis liver (Prussian blue reaction).

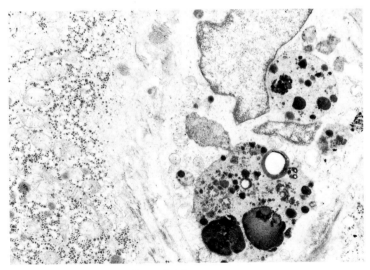

Fig. 125 Electron micrograph of secondary lysosomes.

Exogenous pigmentation

Aetiology   Pigment may enter the body from a variety of sources.

Inhalation

A variety of particles such as coal, stone, asbestos and iron ores may be inhaled and are deposited within the lungs. If excessive then the lungs may be damaged and this is the basis for industrial *pneumoconiosis*. Dust particles of less than 5 μm are taken up by the pulmonary macrophages. The latter may enter the peribronchial lymphatics and the particles are deposited in the respiratory bronchiole walls. Some dusts, e.g. carbon, can accumulate in large amounts and yet cause little damage (*anthracosis*) (Fig. 126), whilst others such as silica can cause severe fibrosis (*silicosis*) (Fig. 127) or may predispose to tumour formation as in *mesothelioma* secondary to asbestos inhalation.

Ingestion

There are now comparatively few ingested pigments. Ingestion of silver-containing medicines imparted a dusky colouration to the skin (*argyria*). In chronic lead poisoning, deposits of lead sulphide give a line of blue pigment around the gums. *Melanosis coli* is secondary to the ingestion of anthracene-based purgatives.

Tattooing

Tattooing in which particles of dyes such as Indian ink, mercuric sulphide and ultramarine are introduced into the epidermis is still practised (Fig. 128). The pigments are permanently deposited; their importance lies not so much in the pigmentation as in the unhygienic methods often employed in tattoo parlours. The main hazard lies in the transmission of viral diseases such as viral hepatitis and AIDS.

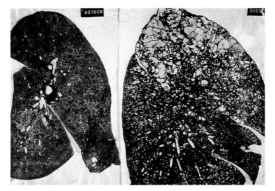

Fig. 126 Anthracosis. (Normal lung on left for comparison.)

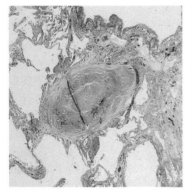

Fig. 127 Silicotic nodules in lung.

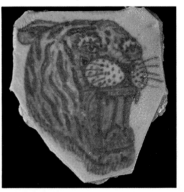

Fig. 128 Tattoo.

25 / **Pathological calcification**

Calcification may occur in the tissues in two main forms: in dystrophic calcification the plasma levels of calcium and phosphate are normal but the tissues in which the calcification occurs are abnormal in some respect; in metastatic calcification abnormally raised levels of plasma calcium result in its deposition in normal tissues.

Dystrophic calcification

Dystrophic calcification may occur in a number of situations:

- In hyalinized dense fibrous tissue as in the walls of aged blood vessels or in those subjected to the effects of raised blood pressure. If severe, the blood vessel wall can be converted into a rigid calcified tube and can be visualized in an X-ray (*Monckeberg's sclerosis*).
- In the dense hyalinized connective tissue of tendons, damaged heart valves (rheumatic or senile) (Fig. 129) and some tumours (e.g. uterine leiomyomas).
- In necrotic tissue, e.g. a caseous lymph node (Fig. 130).
- In inspissated pus which cannot be resolved.
- In old venous thrombi (*phleboliths*) which may be detected in X-rays.
- In organic debris in a variety of situations, such as salivary ducts, kidney and gall bladder, where it may calcify to produce stones (Fig. 131).

Metastatic calcification

Metastatic calcification may be associated with:

- excessive calcium absorption from the gastrointestinal tract as in vitamin D overdose
- conditions in which there is an excess of calcium mobilized from the bones; this can be secondary to bone destruction by tumour or to prolonged immobilization
- primary or secondary hyperparathyroidism.

The calcium is found in the walls of arteries, in the stomach and in the kidneys and lungs.

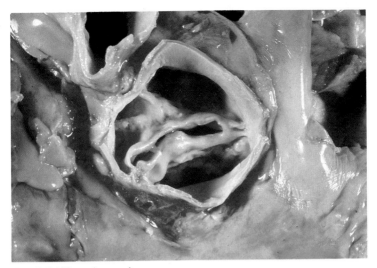

Fig. 129 Calcific aortic stenosis.

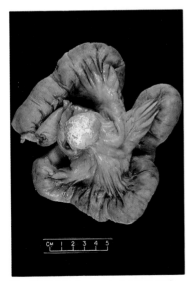

Fig. 130 Calcified mesenteric lymph node (old TB).

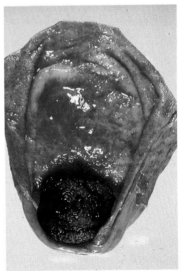

Fig. 131 Gallstone with associated cholecystitis.

26 / Uric acid and urates

Definition Uric acid is the final breakdown product of purines derived from nucleic acids. Some 400 to 700 mg of uric acid is produced daily in an adult and this is largely excreted via the renal distal tubules. Plasma levels are normally maintained below 7 mg/100 ml for men and 6 mg/100 ml for women.

Disorders Raised blood levels of uric acid can be:
- Familial, when they are associated with a deficiency of phosphoribosyl transferase.
- Secondary to increased breakdown of nucleic acids, as in myeloproliferative disorders or leukaemia treated with chemotherapy. Some drugs, including diuretics, and poisons, e.g. lead, interfere with renal excretion of uric acid, which may also be diminished in chronic renal failure. Elevated blood levels are also associated with hyperparathyroidism.

Gross appearance Excess of uric acid and of urates may be deposited in the kidney where they may be seen as a yellowish streaking in the renal medulla and may be associated with chronic renal failure. They may also be deposited in the skin and in and around joints in the condition known as gout. These soft tissue deposits are known as tophi (Fig. 134).

Microscopic appearance The sheaves of crystals so deposited can evoke a marked inflammatory response with a foreign body giant cell reaction (Fig. 133). The needle-shaped crystals are markedly birefringent in polarized light (Fig. 132), and may be detected in aspirates from affected joints.

Historically gout was associated with excess intake of port. Contamination of port wine by bottles made of lead-containing glass is likely to have been responsible for this occurrence.

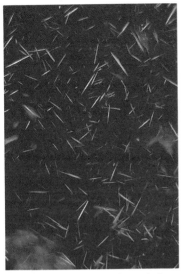

Fig. 132 Urate crystals showing optical birefringence.

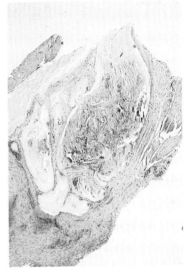

Fig. 133 Gout. Urate crystals with foreign body reaction.

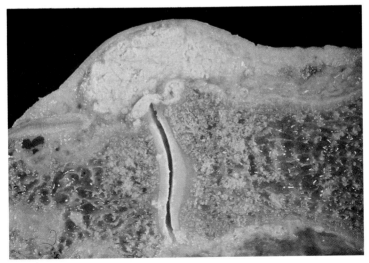

Fig. 134 Gouty tophus in great toe.

27 / Tumours—classification

A tumour or neoplasm is an abnormal mass of cells which grows in an uncontrolled fashion and in which this growth persists after cessation of the initiating stimulus.

Tumours may be classified in two main ways:

- behavioural classification describes the way in which the tumour behaves, i.e. whether it is benign or malignant
- histogenetic classification describes the tumour in terms of its tissue of origin.

Behavioural classification

Various histological and functional characteristics of tumours are used to describe behaviour:

- The *mitotic index* is the proportion of cells seen to be in mitosis (Fig. 135). It is inaccurate as it gives no idea of the cell cycle time.
- Other techniques can assess the proportion of cells entering a particular stage of the cell cycle (*mitotic rate*).
- Loss of cells is a result of cell death caused by abnormal metabolism; ischaemia due to the tumour outgrowing its blood supply shortens cell life span or may cause tumour necrosis (Fig. 136).
- Rapidly growing tumours compress surrounding tissue forming a pseudocapsule (Fig. 137).

The growth rate of a tumour depends on the proportion of cells undergoing mitosis, the duration of the cell cycle and the rate of cell loss.

Malignant tumours are more likely to show these features than benign ones.

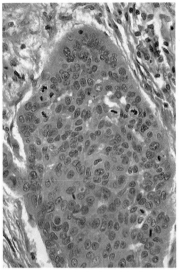

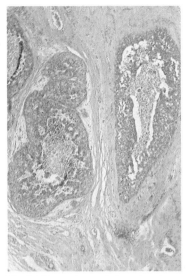

Fig. 135 Increased mitotic activity in a squamous carcinoma.

Fig. 136 Focus of necrosis in an intraduct carcinoma of breast.

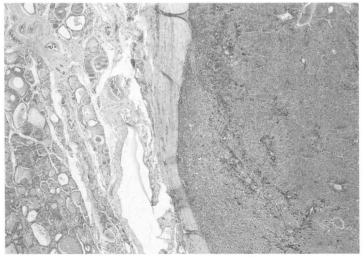

Fig. 137 Pseudocapsule around thyroid adenoma.

Histogenetic classification

Histological differentiation describes how closely the tumour resembles its tissue of origin.

- Variations from normal histological appearances are known as *cellular atypia* or *dysplasia* (the latter term is often used to describe premalignant change in epithelium).
- *Pleomorphism* is variation in cell size and shape, and in the staining characteristics of the cytoplasm and/or nucleus and nucleolus. A high nuclear/cytoplasmic ratio is a typical finding in malignant tumours (Fig. 138).
- *Anaplasia* refers to complete loss of specialized histological features such that the tissue of origin cannot be predicted.

Functional differentiation reflects the tumour cells' ability to reproduce the function (usually secretory) of the cell of origin.

Good differentiation is a feature of benign neoplasms; whereas anaplasia is found in many malignant tumours (Figs 139, 140 & 141).

The ability to transgress the normal tissue boundaries and to invade locally, to penetrate lymphatics and blood vessels and to spread (*metastasize*) to distant sites are the major criteria of malignancy.

Malignant cells must possess the ability to bind to components of the basement membrane, probably by developing laminin receptors; collagenases are then released from the tumour cells and disrupt the basement membrane allowing the tumour cells to enter the matrix surrounding the tumour; further enzymatic digestion allows the tumour cells to migrate through the tissue (p. 133).

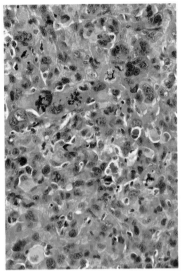

Fig. 138 Pleomorphism of cells in a malignant tumour.

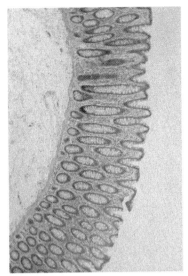

Fig. 139 Normal colonic mucosa.

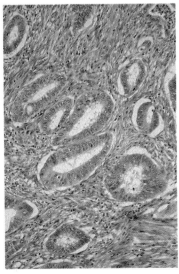

Fig. 140 Well-differentiated colonic adenocarcinoma.

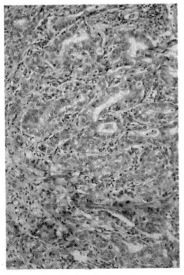

Fig. 141 Anaplastic colonic carcinoma.

Genetic causes

Some neoplasms are associated with identifiable chromosomal alterations.

Retinoblastoma. This rare ocular neoplasm is inherited as an autosomal recessive; both copies of chromosome 13 are deleted.

Burkitt's lymphoma. In Burkitt's lymphoma there is reciprocal translocation of chromosomes 8 and 14, the *c-myc* oncogene being moved adjacent to the immunoglobulin gene on 14, allowing deregulation of the growth of lymphoid cells (see below and Fig. 142).

Chronic myeloid leukaemia. The Philadelphia chromosome (*c-abl* proto-oncogene translocated from chromosome 9 to 22) is a marker for chronic myeloid leukaemia in which the biochemical function of the gene product is altered.

In other inherited neoplasms there are no clearly defined chromosomal abnormalities, e.g. in adenomatosis coli myriads of benign neoplasms develop in the colon and invariably progress to malignant neoplasms.

Oncogenes DNA extracted from certain tumour cells when injected into normal target cells transforms these target cell lines into tumorigenic cells with a transformed phenotype. The transforming ability was shown to be present in certain specific genes— oncogenes—found in the original tumour DNA. Similar genes without the transforming ability— proto-oncogenes—have since been demonstrated in normal cells. Proto-oncogenes may be changed to cellular oncogenes with transforming ability in the process of activation (Fig. 142).

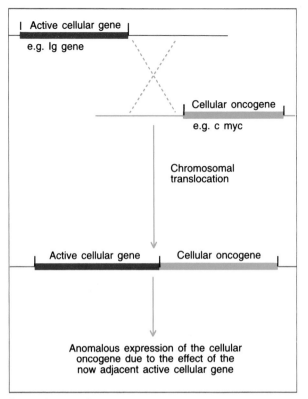

Fig. 142 Diagram of oncogene.

Chemical causes

Percival Pott made the first description of chemical carcinogenesis: scrotal cancer in chimney sweeps. The first experimental evidence for the role of chemicals in the production of tumours was produced in 1915, when Japanese workers used coal tar on rabbit skin.

Multistep theory of carcinogenesis

Most chemical carcinogens require metabolic activation before they react with cells, indicating that cancer is a multistep process (Fig. 143). This metabolic activation is brought about by an initiator, a chemical which causes an irreversible but undetectable change in the cell which then requires a second non-carcinogenic agent, a promoter, to produce the tumour. For example:

- Polycyclic hydrocarbons (benzpyrene, dibenzanthracene) are metabolized by cytochrome P450-dependent oxidases to electrophilic epoxides which react with nucleic acids to cause mutation. Cigarette smoke contains such compounds.
- Aromatic amines and azo dyes are metabolized in the liver and detoxified by glucuronation; hydrolysis in the bladder produces the active hydroxylamine resulting in bladder cancer.
- Nitrosamines have been implicated in gastrointestinal carcinogenesis; they may be produced from nitrates added to food as preservatives.
- Some metals (e.g. Ni^{2+}, Pb^{2+}) are electrophilic and can react with DNA; they may be responsible for some tumours which are associated with specific occupations.

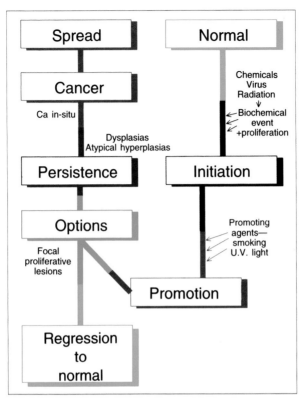

Fig. 143 Diagram of the multistep theory of carcinogenesis.

Physical causes

Ultraviolet radiation

Ultraviolet (UV) radiation (wavelength 290–370 nm) is associated with the development of skin tumours (*basal cell carcinoma, squamous carcinoma, melanocarcinoma*) in white-skinned people exposed to excessive strong sunlight. UV radiation produces pyrimidine dimers which damage the phosphodiester skeleton of DNA. In *xeroderma pigmentosum* (an autosomal recessive condition) there is defective DNA repair, and the UV-induced tumours appear without excessive exposure.

Ionizing radiation

Ionizing radiation is known to cause cancers. It is not known whether there is a threshold dose below which radiation is safe, or whether any exposure is potentially carcinogenic. Thymic irradiation in children resulted in adult thyroid cancer; a radiodiagnostic medium (Thorotrast) was responsible for the development of angiosarcoma of the liver (Fig. 144). The effect of radiation at the cellular level is either acute cell death or mutation.

Asbestos fibres

Asbestos fibres are inhaled (Fig. 145) and, depending on the diameter of the fibre, may reach the periphery of the lung where they produce fibrosis (*asbestosis*), fibrosis of the pleura (*pleural plaques*) and/or a neoplasm (*mesothelioma*) (Fig. 146). The principal type of fibre involved is the long, thin crocidolite. The latent period is 20 years.

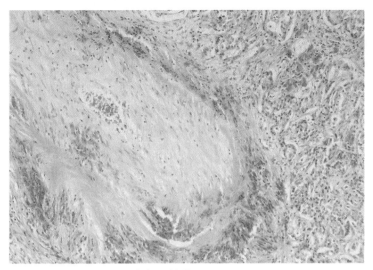

Fig. 144 Angiosarcoma in association with Thorotrast.

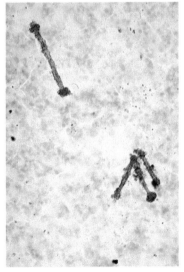

Fig. 145 Asbestos bodies in lung.

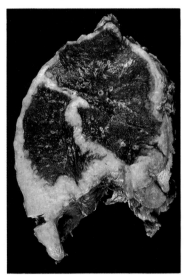

Fig. 146 Mesothelioma in patient exposed to asbestos.

Viral causes

Human papilloma virus (HPV), hepatitis B virus (HBV) and human T-cell leukaemia virus (HTLV1) are associated with human tumours.

DNA viruses DNA viruses contain double-stranded DNA which can be integrated in part or in whole with the host cell chromosomes. They therefore form long-term associations with the host at the cellular level. Persistent or latent infections result and there may be long-term effects on the host genome resulting in neoplasia.

Human papilloma virus. HPV causes benign wart-like lesions on the skin, larynx, vulva and penis. It has been associated with the development of cervical intra-epithelial neoplasia and carcinoma of the cervix, with HPV-DNA integration in host cell DNA being confirmed. There are multiple different types of HPV, type 16 or 18 being most commonly associated with invasive cervical carcinoma (Figs 147 & 148).

Epstein–Barr virus (EBV). This is a herpes virus that transforms B-lymphocytes which have EBV receptors into lymphoblasts and this may progress to Burkitt's lymphoma, particularly in African children (Fig. 149). This virus is also associated with nasopharyngeal carcinoma and some subtypes of Hodgkin's disease.

Cytomegalovirus (CMV). CMV, which is also a herpes virus, may be involved in the production of Kaposi's sarcoma in AIDS patients.

Hepatitis B virus. In areas of high endemic HBV infection there is increased incidence of hepatocellular carcinoma (Fig. 150); the integration of HBV DNA into hepatocyte DNA has been demonstrated.

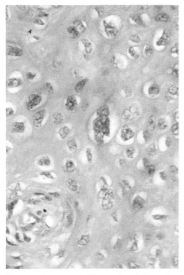

Fig. 147 Human papilloma virus infected cells (koilocytes) in the cervix.

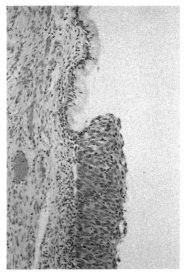

Fig. 148 Cervix showing severe cervical intra-epithelial neoplasia (CIN III).

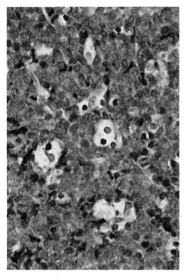

Fig. 149 Burkitt's lymphoma.

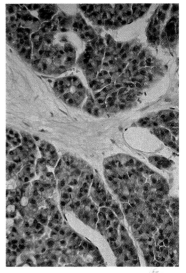

Fig. 150 Hepatocellular carcinoma.

Viral causes (contd)

RNA viruses The only RNA virus confirmed to produce tumours in humans is HTLV1 which produces human T-cell leukaemia/lymphoma. Many tumour-producing RNA viruses are recognized in other animals, some producing tumours in their hosts within a short period of 3 weeks, e.g. the Rous sarcoma virus which contains the *src* transforming gene.

Mechanism of host cell transformation

The discovery of the enzyme reverse transcriptase in 1970 explained how RNA viruses could produce an oncogenic effect.

Viral RNA is transcribed to DNA by reverse transcriptase; this DNA is then integrated into host chromosome DNA.

Acute transforming RNA viruses contain a viral oncogene (Fig. 151) derived by transduction of a cellular proto-oncogene; this viral oncogene is converted to DNA by reverse transcriptase. The DNA copy—the pro-virus—contains the transcribed viral oncogene adjacent to three genes which code for the viral envelope proteins, the viral core proteins and reverse transcriptase. The inserted DNA results in neoplastic transformation in the infected cell.

Long latency RNA viruses do not contain an oncogene but have a promoter gene which deregulates the cellular proto-oncogene (*insertional mutagenesis*).

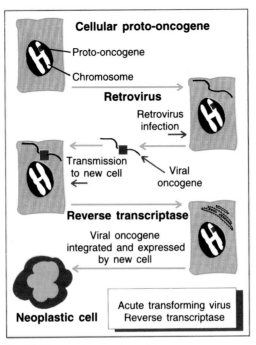

Fig. 151 Diagram of reverse transcriptase.

Hormonal influence

Some tumours are under hormonal influence, and have hormone receptors.

Clinical types

Breast cancer. Breast cancer cells often have oestrogen receptors which may be detected biochemically or by immunocytological techniques (Fig. 152) (p. 131). Receptor-positive cells may respond to anti-oestrogen therapy (tamoxifen—a competitive inhibitor of oestrogen receptor sites). Estimation of oestrogen receptor status may therefore provide an indication of the likelihood of a favourable response (in up to one-third of women) to endocrine therapy.

Prostatic carcinoma. This is under androgenic drive and may respond clinically to either orchidectomy or oestrogen therapy. Thus, after orchidectomy, pain from metastatic lesions may disappear and tumour growth is slowed or halted. Oestrogen therapy is characterized by squamous metaplasia in both benign and malignant prostatic glands; unfortunately the beneficial effect has to be offset against the acceleration of ischaemic heart disease which may occur in the elderly.

Endometrial cancer. This may result from prolonged or unopposed endogenous or exogenous oestrogenic stimulation. There is a spectrum of endometrial changes, from mild hyperplasia through various degrees of atypical change until adenocarcinoma develops. There is a higher incidence of endometrial cancer (Figs 153 & 154) in women with granulosa cell tumours of the ovary which secrete oestrogen.

Vaginal clear cell carcinoma. This occurs in 0.1% of women exposed in utero to diethylstilboestrol (DES). The tumour appears at an early age, usually under 20 years. Many more women exposed to DES develop vaginal adenosis which is benign.

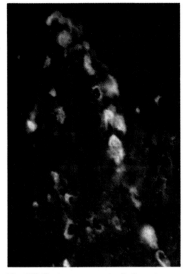

Fig. 152 Oestrogen receptor in breast carcinoma (immunofluorescence).

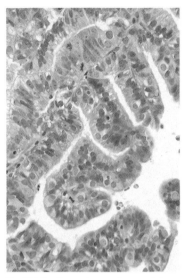

Fig. 153 Papillary adenocarcinoma of the endometrium.

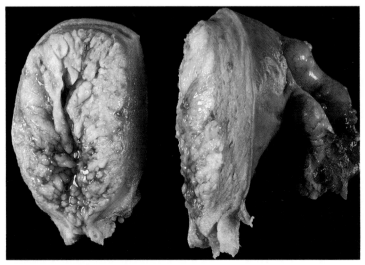

Fig. 154 Endometrial carcinoma.

29 / Tumours—nomenclature

Tumour nomenclature comprises indications of the tumour's derivation and its possible behaviour (pp. 95 & 97).

- *Benign tumours* have the suffix *-oma* which is preceded by an indication of the cell of origin. For example:
  —adenoma = benign tumour of glandular epithelium
  —fibroma = benign tumour of connective tissue.
- *Malignant tumours* use the suffix *-carcinoma* if the tumour is derived from an epithelial source and *-sarcoma* if derived from mesenchyme. For example:
  —adenocarcinoma = malignant tumour of glandular epithelium
  —fibrosarcoma = malignant tumour of connective tissue.

Unfortunately many tumours do not conform to the above rules, their place in the nomenclature being assured by long usage. For example, a *lymphoma* is not a benign proliferation of lymphoid cells but is a malignant tumour.

Benign epithelial tumours

Clinical types **Papillomas**. Benign epithelial tumours derived from surfaces are termed papillomas and consist of fronds (papillae) which are finger-like growths of fibrovascular cores covered by neoplastic epithelium. Papillomas may be sessile or pedunculated.

Adenomas. Tumours derived from solid organs or glandular epithelium are known as adenomas (Figs 155–157). In endocrine organs they are often functionally well differentiated, secreting hormones. In the colon they show various histological patterns and are premalignant.

Cystadenomas. Ovarian tumours are often cystic, and are called cystadenomas. They can be either serous or mucinous depending on their secretory activity.

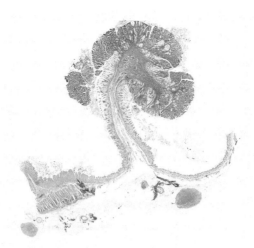

Fig. 155 Tubular adenoma of colon.

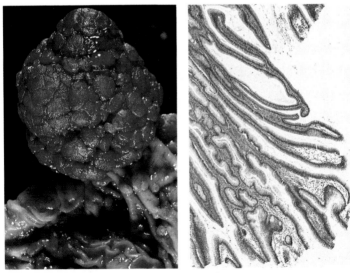

Fig. 156 Tubular adenoma of colon.

Fig. 157 Villous adenoma of colon.

Malignant epithelial tumours

Malignant epithelial tumours are termed *carcinomas* and are the major cause of death from malignant disease. The incidence varies among countries and different tumours predominate in different countries, e.g. gastric carcinoma is common in Japan while lung cancer is very common in Scotland. The reason for these variations may be environmental, genetic, or a combination.

Clinical types

Squamous caricinoma (Fig. 158). This arises from skin, buccal mucosa, pharynx, oesophagus, uterine cervix and at other sites where squamous metaplasia occurs, e.g. bronchus, bladder. The tumour may be well differentiated producing abundant keratin (epithelial pearls) or so poorly differentiated that it becomes spindle-celled, resembling a sarcoma (p. 119).

Adenocarcinomas (Fig. 159). These arise from glandular epithelium and often form acinar or glandular structures which in the better differentiated tumours produce mucins identifiable by the PAS stain. Some adenocarcinomas are solid, infiltrating tumours (e.g. signet-ring cell carcinoma of the stomach) while others may be cystic (e.g. ovarian cystadenocarcinoma); cystic carcinomas are often papillary and these may contain small calcified structures called calcispherites, e.g. thyroid carcinoma.

Transitional cell carcinomas (Fig. 160). These are derived from transitional epithelium: frond-like early tumours progress to solid invasive tumours.

Basal cell carcinoma (rodent ulcers) (Fig. 161). These arise from the sun-exposed areas of skin, usually on the face. Basal cell carcinoma is unusual because it does not metastasize but invades locally, and can be cured by local excision.

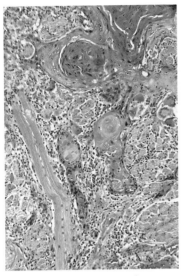

Fig. 158 Squamous carcinoma of tongue.

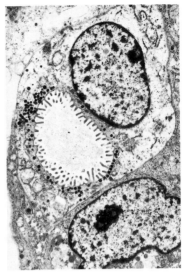

Fig. 159 Adenocarcinoma of breast. Electron micrograph to show intracytoplasmic lumen.

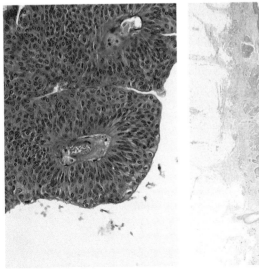

Fig. 160 Transitional cell carcinoma of bladder.

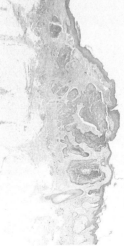

Fig. 161 Basal cell carcinoma of skin.

Malignant epithelial tumours (contd)

Gross appearance
- Carcinoma arising in a solid organ, such as the breast, usually presents as a nodular mass of irregular outline infiltrating the surrounding tissue (Fig. 162).
- Tumours of epithelial surfaces are initially raised nodules which undergo central necrosis producing a crater with raised, rolled margins (Fig. 163).

Microscopic appearance
The gross appearance also reflects the histological features. For example some breast cancers evince a marked fibrous tissue response (*desmoplastic reaction*) and are hard on cutting, e.g. scirrhous carcinoma of breast; others have little connective tissue reaction and are therefore soft to cut—medullary breast carcinoma.

The function of the parent cell may be exaggerated. For example, a mucoid adenocarcinoma of the stomach is characterized by the production of a marked excess of mucin, such that individual tumour cells 'float' in a sea of mucin. In some poorly differentiated adenocarcinomas mucin histochemistry or electron microscopy may be required to demonstrate the few small mucin granules being secreted.

The malignant potential may be assessed by increased mitotic rate, cellular pleomorphism or invasion of blood vessels and/or lymphatics.

Tumour grading
Histological grading involves assessing various features of the tumour which have been shown to affect prognosis. These features are usually ascribed numerical values, such that the highest number implies the worst prognosis. For example, the Bloom and Richardson scheme for ductal breast carcinoma gives a cumulative numerical value to growth pattern, differentiation and mitotic rate.

Tumour staging
In tumour staging attempts are made to combine clinical and pathological prognostic indicators. In the TNM system the local extent of tumour, determined by clinical or pathological examination (T), lymph node involvement (N) and presence of metastases (M) are allocated numerical values.

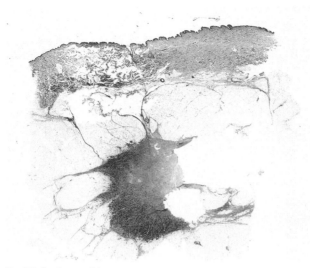

Fig. 162 Carcinoma of breast.

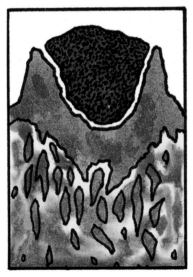

Fig. 163 Diagram of tumour necrosis.

Benign connective tissue tumours

Benign connective tissue tumours produce the matrix associated with the normal tissue. They are usually rounded, well-encapsulated nodules.

Clinical types

Uterine leiomyoma. This consists of interweaving bundles of smooth muscle cells (Fig. 164). Benign smooth muscle tumours may occur in a variety of other sites, e.g. in the wall of the oesophagus or stomach.

Lipoma. This consists of a lobulated mass of adipose tissue usually in the subcutaneous tissue. These may also be found in other sites, e.g. in the wall of the small intestine (Fig. 165).

Chondromas (enchondromas). These are benign cartilage tumours usually arising in the small bones of the hands or feet. They may be multiple, e.g. in Ollier's disease and in Maffucci's syndrome.

Osteomas. These are benign bone-forming tumours. The osteoid osteoma occurs in the shafts of long bones in adolescent males, who complain of nocturnal pain relieved by aspirin.

Fibromas. These are benign tumours of fibrous tissue and whilst they are described in some internal organs, e.g. kidney, they are extremely rare in the soft tissues and may represent reparative processes rather than true neoplasms.

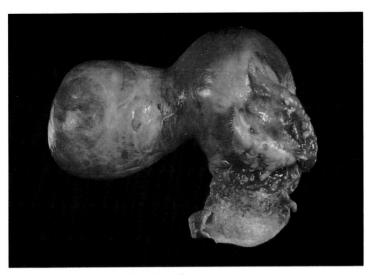

Fig. 164 Leiomyoma (fibroid) of uterine wall.

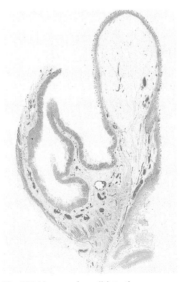

Fig. 165 Lipoma of small intestine.

Malignant connective tissue tumours

Malignant connective tissue tumours are known as *sarcomas*; they are much less common than carcinomas, but are often highly aggressive in their behaviour. Highly vascular, they spread by blood vessel invasion resulting in pulmonary metastases. Although appearing well encapsulated, there is usually local invasion, which means that if the tumour is 'shelled out' by the surgeon, recurrence is inevitable.

Clinical types

Osteosarcoma. This is the commonest sarcoma, arising at the metaphyseal ends of the long bones (Fig. 167). It usually produces recognizable osteoid matrix (Fig. 166). This is usually a tumour of children and young adults. There is a second peak of incidence in the elderly with Paget's disease of bone.

Chondrosarcoma. This arises in the flat bones of an older age group (Fig. 168), or may develop in a chondroma.

Leiomyosarcoma. This occurs in the smooth muscle of the uterus or the wall of the alimentary tract. Differentiation from leiomyoma may be difficult and is dependent on assessment of mitotic activity.

Rhabdomyosarcoma. This develops from skeletal muscle. It is the commonest soft tissue tumour of children and adolescents, but is rare in adults. There are two main types—embryonal and alveolar.

Liposarcoma. This arises in the deep subcutaneous tissue of the trunk, proximal limbs and in the retroperitoneum.

Malignant fibrous histiocytoma. This is the commonest soft tissue sarcoma of adults, arising in the deep soft tissue of the limbs and of the retroperitoneum in those between 50 and 70 years old. This is a highly malignant tumour with a poor prognosis.

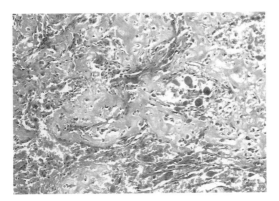

Fig. 166 Osteosarcoma.

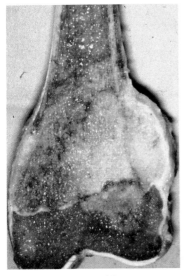

Fig. 167 Osteosarcoma of femur.

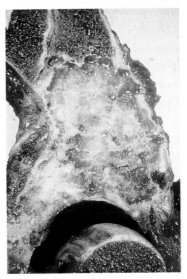

Fig. 168 Chondrosarcoma of pelvis.

Neuroectodermal tumours

Gliomas

These are derived from astrocytes, oligodendrocytes and ependymal cells. Although relatively rare these are the second commonest tumours in children. They cause problems by virtue of their position giving rise to Jacksonian epilepsy, hemiparesis or hemianopia. They may also raise intracranial pressure, in part due to the size of the tumour and in part to surrounding cerebral oedema. The latter responds well to steroid therapy. They do not spread out of the skull.

Astrocytoma. This is the commonest type (Fig. 169). It is usually a poorly defined tumour spreading within the brain. Cystic change is common both grossly and microscopically. Focal areas of anaplasia may occur, indicated by areas of haemorrhage and necrosis.

It is important to note that the commonest tumours within the cranial cavity are metastatic deposits (Fig. 170) and meningiomas (tumours derived from the arachnoid granulations).

Melanocarcinoma (Figs 119 & 120, p. 84)

This usually arises from sun-exposed skin and is characterized by the presence of melanin in the tumour cells. Features suggestive of malignancy in a pigmented lesion include:

- increasing size
- developing itch or inflammation
- irregularity in shape and pigmentation
- the presence of ulceration or bleeding.

It is often a highly malignant tumour, the behaviour being predicted by the depth of invasion of the dermis by the malignant cells. This may be assessed by the Breslow thickness and the Clark level.

The main types are *lentigo maligna*, *superficial spreading*, *nodular* and *acral lentiginous*.

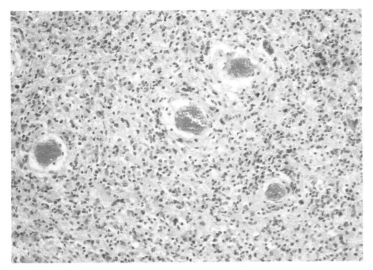

Fig. 169 Astroctyoma.

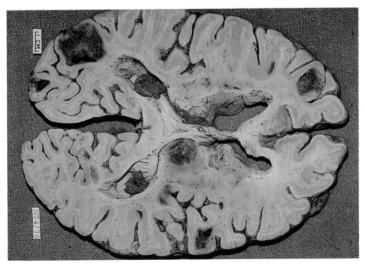

Fig. 170 Pigmented cerebral metastases from a melanocarcinoma.

Haemopoietic tumours

These are derived from the blood cells and are called *leukaemias*. There are many different types arising from various stages of the maturation of lymphocytes or myeloid cells. Occurring in children and adults they may be chronic or acute and are often highly sensitive to chemotherapy.

The acute leukaemias involve proliferation of immature (blast) cells; the chronic forms consist of more mature forms.

Acute leukaemia

Clinical types   There are two main types:
- acute lymphoblastic leukaemia (ALL) (Fig. 171)
- acute non-lymphoblastic leukaemia (ANLL)— myeloid, monocytic, erythroid and megakaryocytic.

ALL is found predominantly in children (80%), while ANLL is a disease predominantly of adults (85%).

Clinically these patients present with recurrent infections, anaemia and bleeding. Diagnosis depends on demonstration of the characteristic blast cells in blood film (Fig. 171) and bone marrow (Fig. 172).

Chronic leukaemia

Clinical types   There are two main types:
- chronic lymphocytic leukaemia (CLL)
- chronic granulocytic leukaemia (CGL).

These are diseases of adults, CLL occurring in the 6th decade, whilst CGL is commonest in the 4th decade.

Large numbers of leucocytes of the appropriate type circulate in the blood and infiltrate the tissues, e.g. the spleen in CLL (Fig. 173). CLL is controlled by drugs in many patients; however, CGL may undergo acute blast transformation as a pre-terminal event.

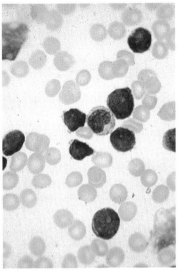

Fig. 171 Blood film of acute lymphoblastic leukaemia.

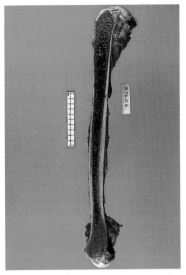

Fig. 172 Extension of red marrow in shaft of femur.

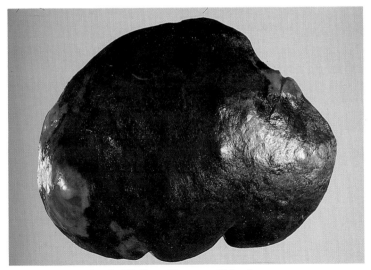

Fig. 173 Enlarged spleen in CLL. Note white areas of infarction.

Lymphoreticular tumours

These are derived from the lymphoid cells of the lymph nodes. There are two major categories, Hodgkin's disease and non-Hodgkin's lymphomas. These are often very sensitive to chemotherapy and may be cured by this means.

Aetiology   The cause of lymphoreticular tumours is unclear but virus infections (e.g. Epstein–Barr virus; Fig. 174) and immunosuppression (e.g. in AIDS) have been implicated.

Clinical types   **Hodgkin's disease.** This is primarily a disease of young adults involving the lymph nodes but extending into extranodal tissues. It is characterized histologically by the presence of the Reed–Sternberg cell—a binucleate cell with mirror-image nuclei and prominent eosinophilic nucleoli (Fig. 175 and Fig. 191, p. 136).

There are four subtypes:

• lymphocyte predominance
• nodular sclerosis
• mixed cellularity
• lymphocyte depletion.

The prognosis also depends on the stage of the disease (Ann-Arbor staging). For example, stage 1 of the disease is confined to one node, whereas in stage 4 there is diffuse involvement of extranodal tissue (Fig. 176).

Non-Hodgkin's lymphoma. These tumours are derived from B- or T-lymphocytes and may be classified according to their immunophenotype. However, their clinical behaviour and prognosis depend more upon their division into low and high grade subtypes. This is determined by the cytology of the main cell type present and by the growth pattern in the lymph node.

• *Low-grade tumours* are characterized by small- to intermediate-sized cells often in a follicular pattern (derived from the B-cells of the germinal centre).
• *High-grade tumours* contain larger cells in a diffuse pattern (derived from germinal centres or from paracortical T-cells) (Fig. 177).

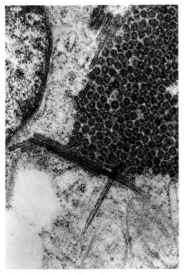

Fig. 174 Epstein–Barr virus.

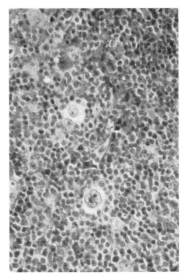

Fig. 175 Mixed cellularity Hodgkin's disease.

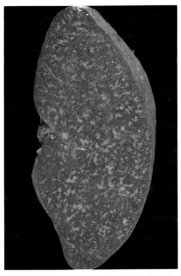

Fig. 176 Spleen—cut surface in Hodgkin's disease.

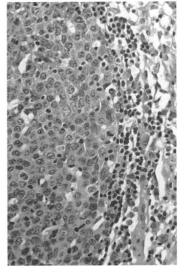

Fig. 177 Follicular lymphoma, centroblastic.

Germ cell tumours

Germ cell tumours are derived from cells of the embryonic germ cell layers. These may occur in both male and female. In the male there are two main types: seminoma and the non-seminomatous germ cell tumours (the majority of which are teratomas).

Definition   A teratoma is composed of tissues derived from the germ cells and contains more than one type of tissue arranged in a totally disorganized fashion. Normally associated with a gonadal origin they may occasionally be found in extragonadal sites, for example mediastinum, pineal gland, retroperitoneum.

Female types   **Dysgerminoma**. This is an undifferentiated germ cell tumour of the ovary which is histologically identical to the seminoma.

Ovarian cystic teratoma (dermoid) (Fig. 178). This is the commonest type in which there are various mature epithelial and connective tissues. This tumour behaves in a benign fashion.

Choriocarcinoma. This arises from placental tissue and secretes chorionic gonadotrophins. This is highly sensitive to methotrexate.

Male types   **Seminoma** (Fig. 179). This testicular tumour occurs in men in their 5th decade. It arises from the testicular tubules and is highly malignant but radiosensitive.

Testicular teratomas (Fig. 180) These tumours which occur in young men are always malignant. They are very complex containing different types of tissue including yolk sac, trophoblast and undifferentiated material. They often secrete substances which can be used as biochemical or immunohistochemical markers for the tumour (alphafetoprotein, HCG). These tumours are sensitive to chemotherapy, particularly to cis-platinum, and the majority of patients can expect to be cured, even after the tumour metastasizes to lymph nodes in the abdomen or thorax.

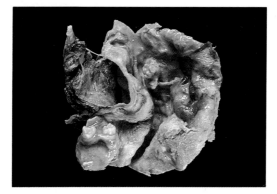

Fig. 178 Ovarian dermoid tumour containing teeth.

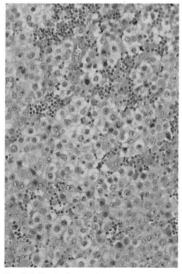

Fig. 179 Testicular seminoma.

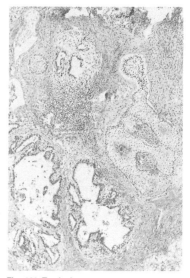

Fig. 180 Testicular teratoma.

Mixed tumours

Occasional tumours contain a mixture of tissue types. This may be the result of:

- collision between two tumours arising in adjacent tissues
- metaplastic changes in a tumour, e.g. endometrial adenosquamous carcinoma.

Some squamous carcinomas may be so dedifferentiated that they become spindle-celled and this mixture of carcinoma and sarcoma in the one tumour is sometimes called (erroneously) a 'carcinosarcoma'.

In some epithelial tumours there are marked stromal changes, e.g. the development of cartilage which gives the appearance of a mixed tumour.

Endocrine tumours

Tissue of origin   **Endocrine**. These tumours regularly produce hormones and often present with the clinical effect of overproduction of the hormone. Tumours derived from the diffuse endocrine system or neuroendocrine system (often termed apudomas or carcinoid tumours; Figs 181 & 182) secrete polypeptide hormones. They may produce multiple hormones, not necessarily those usually associated with the cell of origin of the tumour (ectopic hormone production), e.g. oat cell carcinoma of the lung producing ACTH, and ADH.

Non-endocrine. Other tumours may exhibit inappropriate hormone production from cells of non-endocrine origin. This is presumably due to derepression of genes in the tumour cells resulting in the synthesis of substances not usually secreted by the cell of origin.

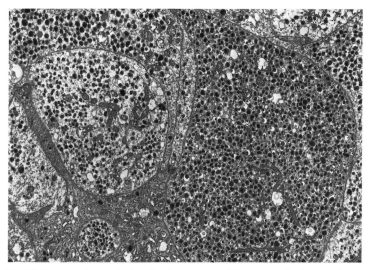

Fig. 181 Electron micrograph of carcinoid tumour containing neuroendocrine granules.

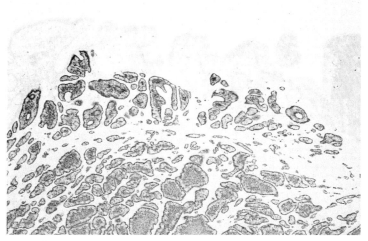

Fig. 182 Carcinoid tumour of small intestine (Grimelius).

30 / Tumour markers

Biochemical markers
Some tumours produce substances which may be detected biochemically in blood or urine, and which may be used in the diagnosis or follow-up of the tumour.

- *Carcinoembryonic antigen* (CEA) was initially thought to be specific for colonic cancer, but is now known to be detectable also in benign bowel diseases, and in other tumours. It may be used in the follow-up of patients after resection of the primary colonic cancer: if the CEA level rises this may indicate recurrence or metastasis.
- *Human chorionic gonadotrophin* (HCG) and *alphafetoprotein* (AFP) are used similarly in teratomas.
- In patients with prostatic carcinoma the serum levels of *prostatic acid phosphatase* (PAP) and *prostate specific antigen* (PSA) can be used in diagnosis and in follow-up.

As yet there is no biochemical marker available for population screening either for malignancy in general or for specific tumour types.

Tissue markers
It is possible to localize substances such as HCG (Fig. 183) or PSA (Fig. 184) in histological tissue sections using immunological techniques (immunocytochemistry) in which antibodies against the marker substance are applied to the tissue section and visualized using immunochemical reagents (Fig. 185).

This technique is useful in determining the broad group of histogenetic origin of an undifferentiated tumour as most tumour cells contain the intermediate filament of their tissue of origin: e.g. carcinomas contain cytokeratins; sarcomas contain vimentin.

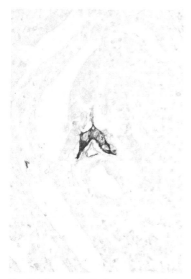

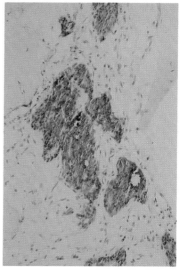

Fig. 183 Human chorionic gonadotrophin in testicular teratoma (immunohistochemistry).

Fig. 184 Prostate adenocarcinoma stained for PSA (immunohistochemistry).

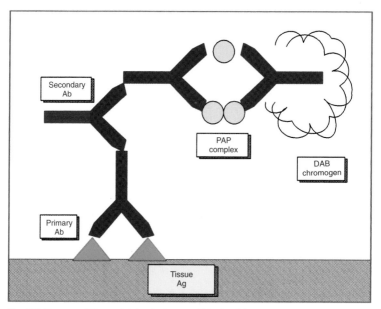

Fig. 185 Diagram of tissue staining by immunohistochemistry.

31 / Spread of tumours

Routes of spread

- Malignant epithelial tumours (carcinomas) spread locally by invasion and permeate lymphatics (Fig. 186); tumour cells travel to lymph nodes and initially colonize the peripheral sinus before replacing the entire node (Fig. 187).
- Veins may be invaded and spread then occurs to the liver (via the portal vein) or lungs (via the vena cava) (Fig. 188).
- Tumours may spread across cavities, e.g. stomach to ovary (Krukenberg tumour).
- Intra-epithelial spread occurs, particularly in the breast, e.g. Paget's disease of the nipple (Fig. 189).
- Retrograde venous spread may occur, e.g. prostatic cancer to the vertebral bodies.
- Malignant connective tissue tumours (sarcomas) are highly vascular and the common route of spread is via the bloodstream, particularly to the lungs ('cannon-ball' secondaries on X-ray).

Mechanisms of invasion

Epithelial tumour cells may produce defective basement membrane substances which fail to arrest growth. In addition many tumour cells produce enzymes which degrade the surrounding extracellular matrix, e.g. proteolytic enzymes including collagenases and cathepsins. They may also produce inhibitors of the normal tissue protease inhibitors. Tumour cells tend to show increased motility and reduced substrate adhesion, contributing to the tumour cell's ability to penetrate the extracellular matrix.

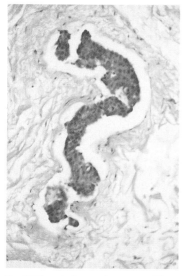

Fig. 186 Lymphatic vessels permeated by tumour.

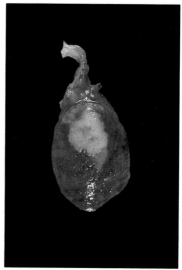

Fig. 187 Metastatic carcinoma in a lymph node. Note afferent lymphatic filled by tumour.

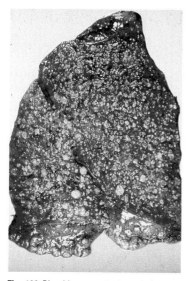

Fig. 188 Blood-borne metastases in lung from a primary renal carcinoma.

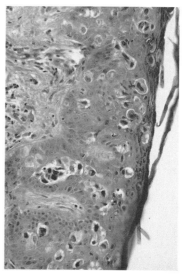

Fig. 189 Paget's disease of the nipple.

32 / Host responses to tumours

Lymphocyte infiltration
Many tumours are associated with a marked infiltrate of lymphoid cells.

- In medullary carcinoma of the breast (Fig. 190) and testicular seminoma, the presence of a large infiltrate of lymphocytes has been associated with a better prognosis.
- In Hodgkin's disease there is a complex mixture of bizarre tumour cells (Reed–Sternberg cells) (Fig. 191), eosinophils, plasma cells and lymphocytes. Those forms of the disease with the least lymphocytes (lymphocyte-depleted Hodgkin's disease) have the worst prognosis.

Rejection
The specific rejection of experimentally transplanted tumours is by T-lymphocytes. Natural killer cells, natural cytotoxic cells and lymphokine-activated killer cells (the latter two stimulated by interleukin-2) may also be involved.

Macrophages
The role of macrophages is unclear. They may kill tumour cells nonspecifically; some macrophage cell products stimulate tumour cell growth and inhibit T-cell reactions.

Antibodies
The role of antibody-dependent, cell-mediated cytotoxicity in killing tumour cells (Fig. 192) is unclear. It is hoped that tagging monoclonal antibodies to tumours with radioactive isotopes or toxins might be useful in treating some tumours.

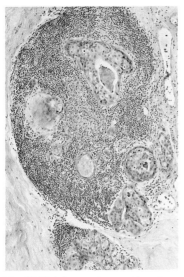

Fig. 190 Medullary carcinoma of breast.

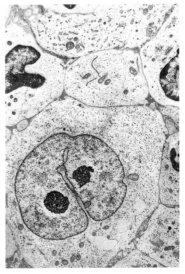

Fig. 191 Hodgkin's disease showing a
Reed–Sternberg cell (electron micrograph).

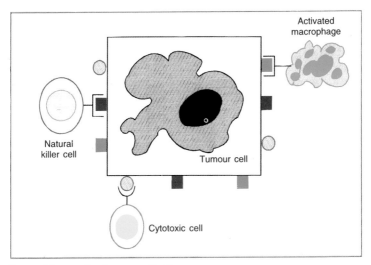

Fig. 192 Diagram of antitumour antibodies.

Index

Abscess in chronic inflammation, 31, 32
Addison's disease, 83
Adenocarcinoma, 113, 114, 115
  breast, 114
  endometrial, 109, 110
  prostatic, 132
Adenoma, 111, 112
  thyroid, 96
Air embolism, 73
Alzheimer's disease, atrophy in, 15, 16
Amyloid, 75-8
Anaplasia, 97, 98
Aneurysms, 67, 68
Angiosarcoma, 103, 104
Anthracosis, 89, 90
Antibodies, antitumour, 135, 136
Arteries
  embolism, 71
  thrombosis, 67
Asbestos, carcinogenicity, 103, 104
Astrocytomas, 121, 122
Atheroma/atheromatous plaque, 71, 72
Atrophy, 15-16
Atypia, cellular, 97
Autolysis, 5-6

Biliverdin/bilirubin, 85
Blood flow
  local reduction, 61-2
  total, changes in, 59-60
Blood vessel, *see* Vasculature
Bone fracture repair, 41-4
Bowel infarction, 61, *see also* Colon
Brain tumours, 121, 122
Breast
  cancer/carcinoma, 96, 109, 110, 114,
    115, 116, 135, 136
  hypertrophy in pregnancy, 49, 50
Bronchitis, chronic, 81, 82
Burkitt's lymphoma, 99, 105, 106

Calcification, pathological, 91-2
Callus, 43, 44
Cancer, *see* Malignant tumour
Capillary thrombosis, 69
Carcinoembryonic antigen, 131
Carcinogenesis, 99-110
Carcinoid tumours, 129, 130
Carcinoma(s), 96, 103, 113-15, *see also*
    Adenocarcinoma; Choriocarcinoma;
    Melanocarcinoma
  breast, 96, 109, 110, 114, 115, 116,
    135, 136
  cervical, 105, 106
  endometrial, 109, 110
  hepatocellular, 105, 106
  metastatic, 133, 134
  mucin production, 81, 82
  prostatic, 109, 110, 131, 132

squamous, 96, 103, 113, 114, 129
  thyroid, medullary, 77
  transitional cell, 113, 114
  vaginal, 109, 110
Cardiac oedema, 55
Cardiogenic shock, 57
Cartilage, repair processes, 45
Caseation, 3, 4
Cell
  damage/injury, 9-14
    by ionizing radiation, 13-14
    non-lethal, 9-12
    repair, *see* Repair
  death
    morphological change with, *see* Necrosis
    programmed, 7-8
Cell cycle, 33, 34
Cerebrum
  infarction, 3, 4, 5, 6
  tumours, 121, 122
Cervical carcinoma, 105, 106
Chemical carcinogens, 101-2
Chemical mediators
  in healing, 33
  in inflammation, 21, 23
Chemotaxis, 23
Chloasma, 83
Chondroma, 117
Chondrosarcoma, 119, 120
Choriocarcinoma, 127
Chorionic gonadotrophin, human, 131, 132
Clot formation, 63, 66, *see also* Coagulation
Coagulation, 63, 64, 65
  activation, 65
  defects, 19
  inhibition, 65
Coagulative necrosis, 3
Collagen in wound healing, 37, 38
Colliquative necrosis, 3
Colon
  adenoma, 111, 112
  carcinoma, 81, 82, 98
Connective tissue
  mucins, 81
  tumours, 117-20, 133
Crohn's disease, 31, 32
Cystadenoma, 111, 112
Cystic fibrosis, 81, 82
Cystic teratoma, ovarian, 127, 128
Cystitis, 27
Cytomegalovirus, 105

Dehydration, 51, 52
Dermoid, 127, 128
Diabetes mellitus, 79
Disseminated intravascular coagulation, 69,
  70
Dysgerminoma, 127
Dystrophic calcification, 91